New Trends in Neuromechanics and Motor Rehabilitation

New Trends in Neuromechanics and Motor Rehabilitation

Editor

Nyeonju Kang

MDPI • Basel • Beijing • Wuhan • Barcelona • Belgrade • Manchester • Tokyo • Cluj • Tianjin

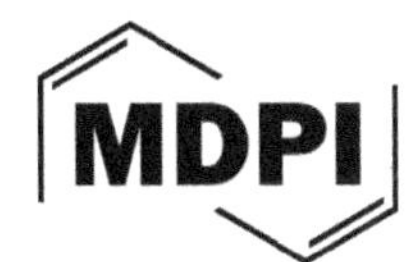

Editor
Nyeonju Kang
Incheon National University
Korea

Editorial Office
MDPI
St. Alban-Anlage 66
4052 Basel, Switzerland

This is a reprint of articles from the Special Issue published online in the open access journal *Applied Sciences* (ISSN 2076-3417) (available at: https://www.mdpi.com/journal/applsci/special_issues/neuromechanics_motor_rehabilitation).

For citation purposes, cite each article independently as indicated on the article page online and as indicated below:

LastName, A.A.; LastName, B.B.; LastName, C.C. Article Title. *Journal Name* **Year**, *Volume Number*, Page Range.

ISBN 978-3-0365-5177-7 (Hbk)
ISBN 978-3-0365-5178-4 (PDF)

Contents

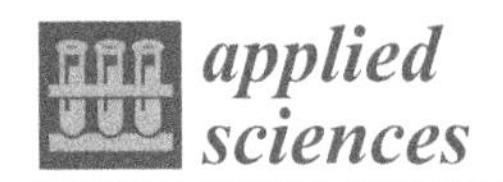
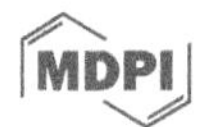

Editorial

Special Issue of New Trends in Neuromechanics and Motor Rehabilitation

Nyeonju Kang

Division of Sport Science, Sport Science Institute & Health Promotion Center, Incheon National University, Incheon 22012, Korea; nyunju@inu.ac.kr

1. Introduction

Neuromechanics has been focused on to investigate both behavioral characteristics and underlying neurophysiological mechanisms for various population, including healthy adults, elderly people, and patients with musculoskeletal and neurological diseases [1]. Moreover, based on cross-sectional findings, researchers can develop new rehabilitation programs that effectively improve behavioral and neurophysiological functions in the motor system. These efforts enable us to identify new neuromechanical outcome measures (e.g., nonlinear measures on EMG signals and force control data) and neuromotor treatments (e.g., non-invasive brain stimulation and functional electrical stimulation).

To summarize and introduce current research topics and tools in the neuromechanical research fields, our Special Issue titled "New Trends in Neuromechanics and Motor Rehabilitation" was launched in 2020, and a total of 10 studies were published. As a guest editor for this Special Issue, I have categorized the published papers in three sections: (a) neuromechanical approaches that characterized motor functions in specific population (six papers), (b) neuromechanical motor rehabilitation techniques (three papers), and (c) comprehensive perspectives in neuromechanical fields (one paper).

2. Neuromechanical Estimation on Motor Functions in Specific Population

For healthy individuals, Clark and Pethick [2] explored side-to-side comparisons (i.e., right/left and dominant/nondominant) of variability and complexity measures that potentially estimate knee muscle force control capabilities. The authors found that only right/left detrended fluctuation analysis (DFA) α, a nonlinear tool, indicated side-to-side difference in uninjured healthy people. These findings suggest that using complexity-based metrics may be a viable option to assess knee neuromuscular control functions in future studies. Min et al. [3] investigated the effects of static stretching and explosive contraction on the quadriceps spinal-reflex excitability and the latency time of the Hoffmann's reflex and motor response. The findings indicated that both static stretching and explosive contraction did not statistically influence the spinal-reflex excitability and the latency time of motor responses. Importantly, the two protocols did not interfere with jumping performances. Overall, these results suggest that either static stretching or explosive contraction can be used for a part of pre-exercise activities.

Following four studies focused on specific population such as people with obesity, children with idiopathic toe walking, elderly people, and older women. Kim et al. [4] determined whether people with obesity differently adapt from treadmill to over-ground walking as compared with people with a normal-weight body mass index. Although both groups showed a transfer of temporal gait adaptation after split-belt treadmill walking, people with obesity showed greater asymmetry for double-limb support time. Potentially, these abnormal adaptation patterns indicated that obesity may influence temporal gait. Soangra et al. [5] examined the hypothesis that typical foot contact dynamics during walking are associated with children diagnosed with Idiopathic Toe walking (cITW) to a higher risk of falling. The authors found that cITW revealed inefficient walking patterns,

Citation: Kang, N. Special Issue of New Trends in Neuromechanics and Motor Rehabilitation. *Appl. Sci.* **2022**, *12*, 7902. https://doi.org/10.3390/app12157902

Received: 31 July 2022
Accepted: 2 August 2022
Published: 6 August 2022

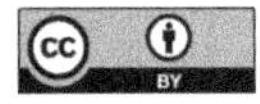

including greater push-off impulses, knee flexion angles, and vertical heel velocity that potentially increase the risk of falls. Lee and Byun [6] performed a pilot study to investigate the effects of aging on postural stability after stepping on a stair. The results indicated that older adults showed greater time to stabilization in the anterior and posterior direction than those for younger adults. These findings suggest that aging may increase the difficulty of dynamic postural control during walking. Kim et al. [7] explored bilateral deficits patterns in late postmenopausal women in their upper extremities. During bilateral and unilateral maximal grip force production tasks, late postmenopausal women revealed greater bilateral deficits (i.e., lower forces during bilateral contraction than the sum of unilateral forces) than those for younger women. The authors posited that age-related muscle weakness and estrogen deficiency may influence bilateral deficits patterns.

3. Neuromechanical Motor Rehabilitation Techniques

Kim et al. [8] determined whether resistance training protocols for upper and lower limbs improve arterial stiffness in healthy young adults, respectively. Their preliminary data found that the resistance training on upper extremities significantly decreased the augmentation index, indicating improved peripheral artery stiffness, and the resistance training on lower extremities showed no significant changes in arterial stiffness. Potentially, providing resistance training for upper extremities may effectively modulate local peripheral artery stiffness even in healthy young adults. To improve muscle functions in adult females with a sedentary lifestyle, Lee et al. [9] used core stabilization exercise programs. For 105 adult females, the exercise intervention improved muscular structural variables of the erector spinae, as indicated by the tensiomyography technique, and further increased functional variables of the muscles during the isokinetic muscular functional test. These findings suggest that the core stabilization exercise effectively decreases stiffness in the erector spinae, as well as isokinetic muscular functions of the trunk. A study performed by Kim and colleagues [10] explored the effects of dance-based aerobic exercise on the affective responses for younger adults with different fitness levels (i.e., sports major and non-major college students). Interestingly, heart rate, responses to the felt arousal scale and the feeling scale were estimated using tailor-made application on a smartwatch. They found that greater affective improvements were observed in the high fit group, suggesting that the level of physical fitness is a crucial factor for the relationship between exercise and affect.

4. Comprehensive Perspectives in Neuromechanical Fields

Cauraugh and Kang [11] conducted a comprehensive narrative review on the topic of bimanual movements and chronic stroke rehabilitation. In a mini-review article, the authors raised the importance of bimanual movement functions in chronic stroke patients because of potential unbalanced cortical activations between hemispheres (i.e., impaired affected hemisphere versus unaffected hemispheres). Specifically, chronic stroke patients showed deficits in kinetic and kinematic control of their upper extremities. Thus, a recovery of the bimanual motor functions can be one of crucial motor rehabilitation goals post stroke. Based on this assumption, many prior studies have focused on activity-based movement treatments, as well as bimanual movement interventions (e.g., bimanual force control practices and bimanual movement actions combined with neuromuscular electrical stimulation) and provided the evidence that patients with stroke revealed improvements in both the bimanual execution and functional recovery of their paretic arm. Taken together, these findings provide a possibility that bimanual movement training protocols in addition to either non-invasive brain stimulation techniques or pharmacological therapies that potentially increase the symmetry of cortical activations between hemispheres.

5. Future Suggestions

The current Special Issue has gathered various scientific approaches to emphasizing neuromechanical tools in cross-sectional research, intervention design, and review studies.

Despite these new findings, an effort to connect altered neurophysiological patterns in the higher center (e.g., brain level) with movement execution is still necessary to further identify new motor control mechanisms in human. Furthermore, biobehavioral science researchers and motor rehabilitation specialists should use various neuromechanical principles to estimate, recover, and understand motor control capabilities in various populations.

Funding: This research received no external funding.

Conflicts of Interest: The author declares no conflict of interest.

References

1. Nishikawa, K.; Biewener, A.A.; Aerts, P.; Ahn, A.N.; Chiel, H.J.; Daley, M.A.; Daniel, T.L.; Full, R.J.; Hale, M.E.; Hedrick, T.L.; et al. Neuromechanics: An integrative approach for understanding motor control. *Integr. Comp. Biol.* **2007**, *47*, 16–54. [CrossRef] [PubMed]
2. Clark, N.C.; Pethick, J. Variability and Complexity of Knee Neuromuscular Control during an Isometric Task in Uninjured Physically Active Adults: A Secondary Analysis Exploring Right/Left and Dominant/Nondominant Asymmetry. *Appl. Sci.* **2022**, *12*, 4762. [CrossRef]
3. Min, K.E.; Lee, Y.; Park, J. Changes in Spinal-Reflex Excitability during Static Stretch and/or Explosive Contraction. *Appl Sci.* **2021**, *11*, 2830. [CrossRef]
4. Kim, D.; Desrochers, P.C.; Lewis, C.L.; Gill, S.V. Effects of Obesity on Adaptation Transfer from Treadmill to Over-Ground Walking. *Appl. Sci.* **2021**, *11*, 2108. [CrossRef]
5. Soangra, R.; Shiraishi, M.; Beuttler, R.; Gwerder, M.; Boyd, L.; Muthukumar, V.; Trabia, M.; Aminian, A.; Grant-Beuttler, M. Foot Contact Dynamics and Fall Risk among Children Diagnosed with Idiopathic Toe Walking. *Appl. Sci.* **2021**, *11*, 2862. [CrossRef]
6. Lee, H.; Byun, K. Postural Instability after Stepping on a Stair in Older Adults: A Pilot Study. *Appl Sci.* **2021**, *11*, 1885. [CrossRef]
7. Kim, J.S.; Hwang, M.H.; Kang, N. Bilateral Deficits during Maximal Grip Force Production in Late Postmenopausal Women. *Appl. Sci.* **2021**, *11*, 8426. [CrossRef]
8. Kim, M.; Lee, R.; Kang, N.; Hwang, M.H. Effect of Limb-Specific Resistance Training on Central and Peripheral Artery Stiffness in Young Adults: A Pilot Study. *Appl. Sci.* **2021**, *11*, 2737. [CrossRef]
9. Lee, H.; Kim, C.; An, S.; Jeon, K. Effects of Core Stabilization Exercise Programs on Changes in Erector Spinae Contractile Properties and Isokinetic Muscle Function of Adult Females with a Sedentary Lifestyle. *Appl. Sci.* **2022**, *12*, 2501. [CrossRef]
10. Kim, Y.; Kim, J.; Woo, M. The Pattern of Affective Responses to Dance-Based Group Exercise Differs According to Physical Fitness, as Measured by a Smartwatch. *Appl. Sci.* **2021**, *11*, 1540. [CrossRef]
11. Cauraugh, J.H.; Kang, N. Bimanual Movements and Chronic Stroke Rehabilitation: Looking Back and Looking Forward. *Appl. Sci.* **2021**, *11*, 858. [CrossRef]

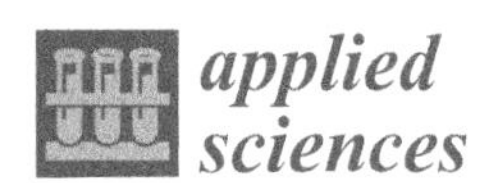

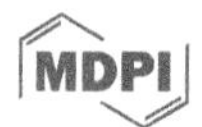

Article

Variability and Complexity of Knee Neuromuscular Control during an Isometric Task in Uninjured Physically Active Adults: A Secondary Analysis Exploring Right/Left and Dominant/Nondominant Asymmetry

Nicholas C. Clark * and Jamie Pethick

School of Sport, Rehabilitation, and Exercise Sciences, University of Essex, Wivenhoe Park, Colchester CO4 3SQ, UK; jp20193@essex.ac.uk
* Correspondence: n.clark@essex.ac.uk

Abstract: Work is needed to better understand the control of knee movement and knee health. Specifically, work is needed to further understand knee muscle force control variability and complexity and how it is organized on both sides of the body. The purpose of this study was to explore side-to-side comparisons of magnitude- and complexity-based measures of knee muscle force control to support future interpretations of complexity-based analyses and clinical reasoning in knee injury control. Participants (male/female n = 11/5) performed constant-force isometric efforts at 50% maximal effort. Force variability was quantified during the constant-force efforts using a coefficient of variation (CV%) and force complexity using approximate entropy (ApEn) and detrended fluctuation analysis (DFA) α. Outcomes were right/left and dominant/nondominant group-level and individual-level comparisons. A limb-symmetry index was calculated for each variable and clinically significant absolute asymmetry was defined (>15%). The only significant side-to-side difference was for right/left DFA α ($p = 0.00$; $d = 1.12$). Maximum absolute asymmetries were (right/left, dominant/nondominant): CV 18.2%, 18.0%; ApEn 34.5%, 32.3%; DFA α 4.9%, 5.0%. Different side-to-side comparisons yield different findings. Consideration for how side-to-side comparisons are performed (right/left, dominant/nondominant) is required. Because a significant difference existed for complexity but not variability, this indicates that both complexity-based and magnitude-based measures should be used when studying knee muscle force control.

Keywords: knee; neuromuscular control; force control; variability; complexity; asymmetry

Citation: Clark, N.C.; Pethick, J. Variability and Complexity of Knee Neuromuscular Control during an Isometric Task in Uninjured Physically Active Adults: A Secondary Analysis Exploring Right/Left and Dominant/Nondominant Asymmetry. *Appl. Sci.* **2022**, *12*, 4762. https://doi.org/10.3390/app12094762

Academic Editor: Nyeonju Kang

Received: 31 March 2022
Accepted: 7 May 2022
Published: 9 May 2022

1. Introduction

The knee accounts for 46.8% of musculoskeletal injuries [1] with ligament and meniscus injuries being frequent [2]. The consequences of knee injury include physical disability [3], substantial healthcare costs [4], and post-trauma osteoarthritis [5]. Therefore, the exploration of factors affecting the control of knee movement and health is necessary for informing knee injury control interventions that support individuals' lifelong physical activity.

Injury control involves the prevention, acute care, and rehabilitation phases of healthcare [6]. When considering aspects of knee movement and health, clinicians make side-to-side comparisons of knee characteristics (e.g., right/left, dominant/nondominant) [7,8]. The reasoning for a right/left or dominant/nondominant side-to-side comparison should be considered carefully because one can yield different findings to the other [9] and because limb dominance changes according to the nature of the task (e.g., muscle strength vs. skill) [10]. Regardless of whether a right/left or dominant/nondominant side-to-side comparison is performed, the premise of a side-to-side comparison is that one side represents a reference standard for clinical judgments relative to the opposite side [7,11]. Therefore, before a valid clinical judgment can be made in injury control as a result of comparing one side to the opposite side, exploratory research is needed to first understand biological phenomena and provide reference data from uninjured individuals [12]. The side-to-side comparison of a variable is termed a "symmetry analysis" [13]; symmetry exists when a variable is equal in magnitude for both limbs and asymmetry exists when a variable is unequal in magnitude for both limbs [14]. In knee injury control, symmetry analyses are performed frequently using variables representing aspects of knee neuromuscular control.

In joint injury control, neuromuscular control refers to the activation of the dynamic restraints (skeletal muscles) in preparation for and response to joint loading and motion to maintain functional joint stability [15]. One aspect of neuromuscular control that has received little attention with regard to symmetry analysis is muscle force control. Physiological signals, such as muscle force, represent interactions between multiple physiological components and asynchronous feedback loops operating over a range of temporal and spatial scales and are characterized by constant fluctuations in system output [16]. The quantification of fluctuations in muscle force signals is, therefore, necessary to better analyze knee neuromuscular control characteristics. The behavior of physiological signals can be analyzed using measures of variability or complexity [17,18]. Metrics of variability are linear and magnitude-based (e.g., standard deviation [SD], coefficient of variation [CV]; Figure 1, *y*-axis) [19,20]. Metrics of complexity are nonlinear and time-based (e.g., approximate entropy, detrended fluctuation analysis; Figure 1, *x*-axis) [21,22]. Specifically, complexity metrics characterize moment-to-moment relationships between successive data points, thereby examining how a signal's structure changes over time (Figure 1, *x*-axis) [17,20]. Magnitude-based measures cannot quantify temporal irregularities and, therefore, miss "hidden information" regarding signal fluctuations [17]. Subsequently, several authors have used complexity analyses (nonlinear time-series analyses) for studying different aspects of human movement in order to gain more information and understanding of the control of posture [23], balance [24], and walking gait [25].

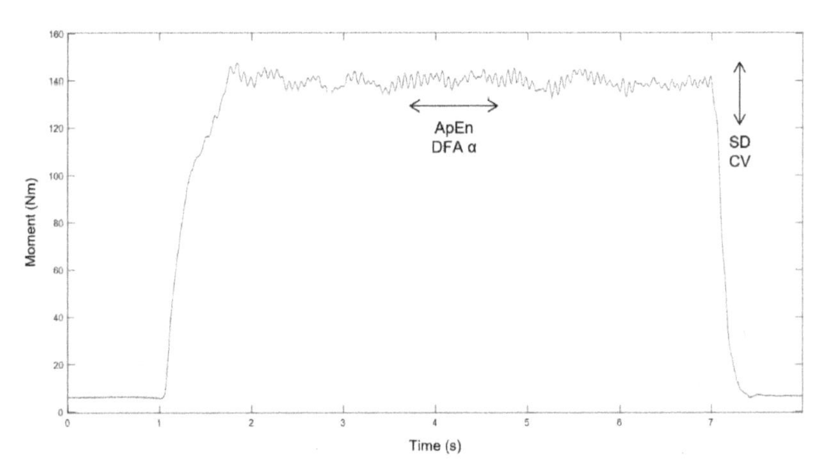

Figure 1. Illustration of how variability-based (magnitude-domain, *y*-axis) and complexity-based (time-domain, *x*-axis) variables relate to the graphical plot of an isometric knee extension signal. Nm = Newton-meters; s = seconds; SD = standard deviation; CV = coefficient of variation; ApEn = approximate entropy; DFA α = detrended fluctuation analysis α. See Methods for explanation of ApEn and DFA α.

Complex fluctuations in physiological processes represent the range across which biological systems function and their ability to respond to unpredictable environments [16]. Complex fluctuations in neuromuscular control reflect the ability to adapt motor output rapidly and accurately in response to task demands [26]. In knee neuromuscular control, some researchers have used magnitude-based metrics [27], others have used complexity-based metrics [20], but few have used both magnitude- and complexity-based metrics [28]. No published work reports examining knee neuromuscular control using both magnitude- and complexity-based measures within both right/left and dominant/nondominant side-to-side analyses in uninjured individuals. Therefore, there is a gap in the literature for exploratory analyses into knee muscle force control variability and complexity and how it is organized specifically on both sides of the body.

The supplementary (secondary) analysis of primary data fulfills a valuable role in scientific inquiry and is encouraged to facilitate research economy, answer interdisciplinary research questions, and mitigate research waste [29,30]. Secondary analysis can be undertaken at any stage of a research project and is further encouraged where primary data from relatively "small-scale experiments" is used to build a foundation for planning future larger-scale original studies and plot a direction for new basic and applied research questions [31]. Accordingly, this study was a secondary analysis of data collected for a prior project [32,33]. The first purpose was to test the hypothesis that there would be no statistically-significant side-to-side differences (right/left, dominant/nondominant) for magnitude- and complexity-based variables extracted from isometric knee extension sub-maximal force output during a constant-force task. The second purpose was to test the hypothesis that the mean side-to-side (right/left, dominant/nondominant) absolute-asymmetry for the magnitude- and complexity-based variables using the limb symmetry index (LSI) would be $\leq$15%; this hypothesis was based on previous research on knee extension neuromuscular control with uninjured individuals [34]. The present exploratory analyses are practically significant because they provide new preliminary reference data that helps to better understand the control of knee movement for both sides of the body in uninjured individuals; these findings will, in turn, inform and support the design and direction of future larger-scale primary studies of motor control and knee health in uninjured and injured individuals.

2. Materials and Methods

2.1. Study Design, Ethical Approval, Informed Consent, Participants

This study was a secondary analysis of data collected for a larger research project [32,33]. Ethics approval was obtained for the original work. Informed consent was provided by all participants. For the original project, inclusion criteria were physically-active males/females aged 18–40 years, and exclusion criteria were current lower limb pain and any lower limb injury in the previous three months. Sixteen participants were available from the original datasets (11 male, 5 female; mean $\pm$ SD: age 24.0 $\pm$ 5.3 years; height 1.74 $\pm$ 0.08 m; body mass 68.3 $\pm$ 11.1 kg).

2.2. Original Experimental Procedures

Participants attended the laboratory on three occasions with $\geq$48 h between sessions. Participants were instructed to avoid any fatiguing exercise/sports for 24 h beforehand. During the first session, participants were familiarized with the instrumentation and procedures, their dynamometer settings were recorded, and limb dominance was established (preferred leg to kick a football). For the next two sessions, isometric knee extension efforts were performed and data were collected for all variables. Limb order was randomized, with one limb assessed in session 2 and the opposite limb assessed in session 3.

2.3. Dynamometry

Isometric knee extension efforts were sampled with a CSMi isokinetic dynamometer (HUMAC Norm, Stoughton, MA, USA), initialized and calibrated according to the manufacturers' instructions. Participants sat with their hips and knees flexed 85° and 90°, respectively, and the lateral epicondyle of the knee aligned with the axis of rotation of the dynamometer lever-arm. The trunk and pelvis were secured using the device's straps. The lever arm's attachment was adjusted so the lower edge of the shin pad was just above the malleoli. The sampling frequency was 1000 Hz.

2.4. Isometric Knee Extension Efforts

Participants performed a series of 3-s maximal voluntary efforts (MVE) separated by 60 s of rest and which continued until the peak moment in three consecutive efforts were within 5% of each other. Participants then performed a 50% MVE constant-force task, with this target based on the peak knee extension moment identified during the MVEs. A chart containing the instantaneous knee extension moment was projected onto a screen placed ~1 m in front of the participant. A scale consisting of a 1 mm thick line was superimposed on the chart and acted as a target so that participants were able to match their instantaneous moment to the target during each trial. Participants were instructed to match their instantaneous moment with the target superimposed on the display for as much of each trial as possible. Five trials were performed, each lasting six seconds and separated by four seconds of rest.

2.5. Data Acquisition and Reduction

Devices were connected by BNC cables (Digitimer, Welwyn Garden City, UK) to a Biopac MP150 and a CED Micro 1401-3 (Cambridge Electronic Design, Cambridge, UK) interfaced with a personal computer. Data were collected in Spike2 software (Version 7, Cambridge Electronic Design, Cambridge, UK). Raw data were processed using customized code in MATLAB R2017a (Mathworks, Natick, MA, USA).

For all variability and complexity analyses, the steadiest five seconds of each 50% MVE trial was identified as the five-second epoch with the lowest SD [20]. Variability and complexity were, therefore, analyzed using 5000 data points. The CV was used as a magnitude-based variable, representing force variability normalized to the mean force [20]. Multiple complexity metrics are recommended for probing subtly different aspects of physiological signals [21]. Approximate entropy (ApEn) [22] was used to determine the regularity/randomness of the force signal and temporal fractal scaling was estimated using detrended fluctuation analysis (DFA) α [35]. Sample entropy [36] was also considered; however, as shown by Pethick et al. [20], this measure does not differ from muscle force ApEn when 5000 data points are used in their calculation. The full details of the calculation of ApEn and DFA α can be found in Pethick et al. [20].

In short, ApEn quantifies the negative natural logarithm of the conditional probability that a template of length m is repeated during a time series. If the data are highly regular, then templates similar for m points (within the tolerance r) are likely to be similar for $m + 1$ points. In this situation, the conditional probability will be close to 1, and the negative logarithm, and therefore the entropy, will be close to zero. This reflects low complexity and high predictability. ApEn was calculated with the template length, m, set at two and the tolerance, r, set at 10% of the SD of knee extension moment output [20,37]; 10% was chosen over other percentages following the recommendations of Forrest et al. [37], who sought to identify a "gold standard" for signal acquisition and processing parameters in the context of the ApEn analyses of isometric muscle force control records. In the DFA algorithm, the time-series of interest is integrated, then divided into boxes of equal length, n, and a least-squares line (representing the trend in each box) is fitted. The integrated time series is detrended by subtracting the local trend in each box, and the root mean square of this integrated, detrended series, $F(n)$, is calculated. This calculation is then repeated over all timescales or box sizes. The slope of the line relating $\log F(n)$ to $\log n$ determines the DFA α scaling exponent [21]. Subsequently, DFA was calculated using 57 boxes, ranging from 1250 to 4 data points. The log-log plot of fluctuation size versus box size was plotted for each participant to identify any significant crossover (as shown by an $r < 0.95$) and the presence of two trends [38]. No cases of significant crossover were observed. Typically, DFA α ranges from ~0.5 to ~1.5 and acts as an indicator of the "roughness" of the time series; the larger the value of α, the more regular the time series [21].

2.6. Statistical Analyses

The mean CV, ApEn, and DFA α from the five 50% MVE constant-force trials were used for analyses. Summary statistics were calculated, including the absolute side-to-side differences (right–left, dominant–nondominant). The minus sign was removed from negative differences.

For statistical analyses (group-level), the normality of data was assessed with histogram inspection and Shapiro–Wilk tests. Alpha was set *a priori* at 0.05. Bonferroni-corrected paired *t*-tests were used for right/left and dominant/nondominant side-to-side comparisons across all variables. Ninety-five percent confidence intervals (CI) were estimated for all variables and within-group Cohen's *d* was calculated for all side-to-side comparisons; effect sizes of 0.20, 0.50, and 0.80 were considered small, medium, and large, respectively [12].

For clinical analyses (individual-level), two LSIs were calculated: right/left LSI (R/L-LSI) [13] and dominant/nondominant LSI (D/ND-LSI). The R/L-LSI (%) was calculated: (right ÷ left) × 100 [13]. A R/L-LSI of 100% represented side-to-side symmetry, <100% lower right-side/higher left-side values, >100% lower left-side/higher right-side values. The D/ND-LSI (%) was calculated: (dominant ÷ nondominant) × 100. A D/ND-LSI of 100% represented side-to-side symmetry, <100% lower dominant-side/higher nondominant-side values, >100% lower nondominant-side/higher dominant-side values. Therefore, for the R/L-LSI and D/ND-LSI, each indicated both the magnitude and direction of asymmetry [13]. Because the size of an absolute asymmetry is frequently the principal matter of clinical interest [13], the absolute asymmetry for both the R/L-LSI and D/ND-LSI was calculated: 100%—participant's LSI [13]. Minus signs were removed from negative differences [13].

3. Results

Summary statistics are presented for the CV in Table 1, ApEn in Table 2, and DFA α in Table 3. All data were normally distributed.

Table 1. Summary statistics and effect sizes for the coefficient of variation (n = 16).

	CV (%)			CV (%)		
	R	L	R-L Absolute Diff.	D	ND	D-ND Absolute Diff.
Min	2.01	2.28	0.02	2.22	2.01	0.02
Max	3.51	6.20	3.64	3.51	6.20	3.64
95% CI	2.53, 2.96	2.67, 3.82	0.20, 1.22	2.54, 2.93	2.68, 3.83	0.20, 1.22
Mean	2.75	3.24	0.71	2.74	3.25	0.71
SD	0.40	1.07	0.96	0.37	1.08	0.96
ES	0.45			0.47		

CV = coefficient of variation; R = right; L= left; R-L Absolute Diff. = right − left (+/− sign removed); D = dominant; ND = nondominant; D-ND Absolute Diff. = dominant − nondominant (+/− sign removed); Min = minimum; Max = maximum; 95% CI = 95% confidence interval (lower bound, upper bound); SD = standard deviation; ES = effect size.

Table 2. Summary statistics and effect sizes for approximate entropy (n = 16).

	ApEn			ApEn		
	R	L	R-L Absolute Diff.	D	ND	D-ND Absolute Diff.
Min	0.25	0.14	0.01	0.25	0.14	0.01
Max	0.65	0.54	0.29	0.65	0.62	0.29
95% CI	0.37, 0.50	0.31, 0.42	0.06, 0.14	0.34, 0.46	0.33, 0.46	0.06, 0.14
Mean	0.43	0.36	0.10	0.40	0.39	0.10
SD	0.12	0.10	0.07	0.11	0.13	0.07
ES	0.73			0.08		

ApEn = approximate entropy; R = right; L= left; R-L Absolute Diff. = right − left (+/− sign removed); D = dominant; ND = nondominant; D-ND Absolute Diff. = dominant − nondominant (+/− sign removed); Min = minimum; Max = maximum; 95% CI = 95% confidence interval (lower bound, upper bound); SD = standard deviation; ES = effect size.

Table 3. Summary statistics and effect sizes for detrended fluctuation analysis α (n = 16).

	DFA α			DFA α		
	R	L	R-L Absolute Diff.	D	ND	D-ND Absolute Diff.
Min	1.17	1.26	0.00	1.26	1.17	0.00
Max	1.52	1.62	0.21	1.56	1.62	0.21
95% CI	1.33, 1.47	1.40, 1.50	0.04, 0.99	1.36, 1.45	1.38, 1.49	0.41, 0.99
Mean	1.38 [a]	1.45	0.07	1.40	1.43	0.07
SD	0.10	0.09	0.06	0.09	0.11	0.06
ES	1.12			0.34		

DFA α = detrended fluctuation analysis α; R = right; L= left; R-L Absolute Diff. = right − left (+/− sign removed); D = dominant; ND = nondominant; D-ND Absolute Diff. = dominant − nondominant (+/− sign removed); Min = minimum; Max = maximum; 95% CI = 95% confidence interval (lower bound, upper bound); SD = standard deviation; ES = effect size; [a] = significant side-to-side difference, $p = 0.00$.

Example findings from the 50% MVE constant-force task for two different participants are illustrated in Figures 2 and 3. The only significant side-to-side differences were for the right/left DFA α ($p = 0.00$; Table 3). For effect sizes, a little under large effect was evident for right/left ApEn (Table 2). A very large effect was evident for right/left DFA α (Table 3).

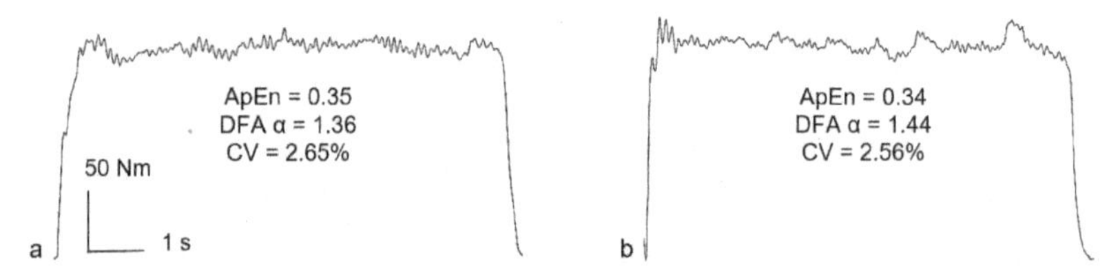

Figure 2. Raw output from a trial for a participant with similar complexity and variability values on the right (**a**) and left (**b**) sides. Nm = Newton-meters; s = seconds; ApEn = approximate entropy; DFA α = detrended fluctuation analysis α; CV = coefficient of variation. ApEn right/left limb-symmetry-index = 102.9%; ApEn right/left absolute-asymmetry = 2.9%. DFA α right/left limb-symmetry-index = 94.4%; DFA α right/left absolute-asymmetry = 5.6%. CV right/left limb-symmetry-index = 103.5%; CV right/left absolute-asymmetry = 3.5%.

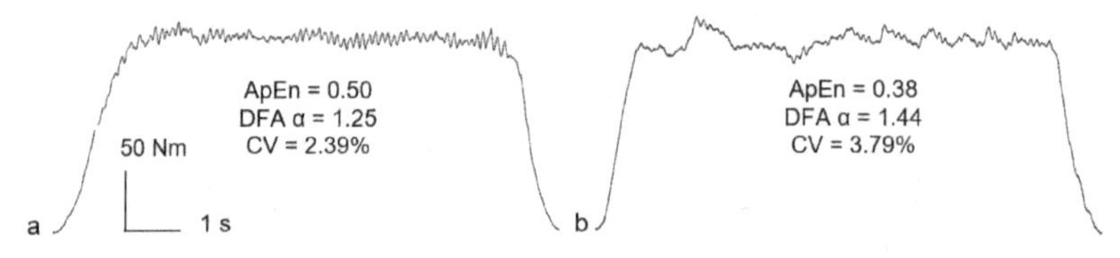

Figure 3. Raw output from a trial for a participant with different complexity and variability values on the right (**a**) and left (**b**) sides. Nm = Newton-meters; s = seconds; ApEn = approximate entropy; DFA α = detrended fluctuation analysis α; CV = coefficient of variation. ApEn right/left limb-symmetry-index = 131.6%; ApEn right/left absolute-asymmetry = 31.6%. DFA α right/left limb-symmetry-index = 86.8%; DFA α right/left absolute-asymmetry = 13.2%. CV right/left limb-symmetry-index = 63.1%; CV right/left absolute-asymmetry = 36.9%.

Summary statistics for R/L-LSIs, D/ND-LSIs, and absolute asymmetries are presented in Tables 4–6. The mean absolute-asymmetry values for both side-to-side comparison methods were >15% for CV and ApEn (Tables 4 and 5). The inspection of the maximum absolute-asymmetry values for both side-to-side comparison methods demonstrates some participants had very large absolute-asymmetries for the CV and ApEn (Tables 4 and 5).

Table 4. Summary statistics for the coefficient of variation limb symmetry indices and absolute asymmetries (n = 16).

	CV		CV	
	R/L Limb Symm. Index (%)	R/L Absolute Asymm. (%)	D/ND Limb Symm. Index (%)	D/ND Absolute Asymm. (%)
Min	41.2	0.7	41.2	0.7
Max	131.2	58.8	120.7	58.8
95% CI	78.3, 102.3	9.7, 26.7	78.2, 101.7	9.7, 26.4
Mean	90.3	18.2	90.0	18.0
SD	22.6	16.0	22.0	15.7

CV = coefficient of variation; R/L = right/left; D/ND = dominant/nondominant; Limb Symmetry Index, see text for equation and explanation; Absolute Asymmetry, see text for equation and explanation; Min = minimum; Max = maximum; 95% CI = 95% confidence interval (lower bound, upper bound); SD = standard deviation.

Table 5. Summary statistics for approximate entropy symmetry indices and absolute asymmetries (n = 16).

	ApEn		ApEn	
	R/L Limb Symm. Index (%)	R/L Absolute Asymm. (%)	D/ND Limb Symm. Index (%)	D/ND Absolute Asymm. (%)
Min	58.3	2.4	58.3	2.4
Max	309.6	209.6	309.6	209.6
95% CI	99.6, 156.1	8.5, 60.4	83.2, 144.2	6.4, 58.2
Mean	127.9	34.5	113.7	32.3
SD	53.0	48.6	57.2	48.6

ApEn = approximate entropy; R/L = right/left; D/ND = dominant/nondominant; Limb Symmetry Index, see text for equation and explanation; Absolute Asymmetry, see text for equation and explanation; Min = minimum; Max = maximum; 95% CI = 95% confidence interval (lower bound, upper bound); SD = standard deviation.

Table 6. Summary statistics for detrended fluctuation analysis α symmetry indices and absolute-asymmetries (n = 16).

	DFA α		DFA α	
	R/L Limb Symm. Index (%)	R/L Absolute Asymm. (%)	D/ND Limb Symm. Index (%)	D/ND Absolute Asymm. (%)
Min	86.8	0.3	86.8	0.3
Max	101.7	13.2	108.1	13.2
95% CI	93.2, 97.7	3.0, 6.9	94.9, 101.4	3.0, 7.0
Mean	95.5	4.9	98.2	5.0
SD	4.2	3.7	6.1	3.7

DFA α = detrended fluctuation analysis α; R/L = right/left; D/ND = dominant/nondominant; Limb Symmetry Index, see text for equation and explanation; Absolute Asymmetry, see text for equation and explanation; Min = minimum; Max = maximum; 95% CI = 95% confidence interval (lower bound, upper bound); SD = standard deviation.

4. Discussion

The first purpose of this study was to test the hypothesis that there would be no statistically-significant side-to-side differences (right/left, dominant/nondominant) for magnitude- and complexity-based variables during an isometric knee extension 50% MVE constant-force task. The only significant difference in either comparison was for right/left DFA α (Table 3). The second purpose of this study was to test the hypothesis that the mean side-to-side (right/left, dominant/nondominant) absolute-asymmetry for the magnitude- and complexity-based variables, assessed using the LSI, would be $\leq$15% for both side-to-side comparisons. The mean absolute-asymmetry was >15% for both comparisons for CV and ApEn (Tables 4 and 5), but not for either comparison for DFA α (Table 6).

In knee health and injury control, side-to-side comparisons inform clinical reasoning and support clinical decision-making [7,13]. At the group level, symmetry analyses examine whether statistically significant side-to-side differences exist for measures of central tendency [13]. The only significant side-to-side group-level differences were for right/left DFA α (Table 3). Interestingly, the significant finding was for a right/left comparison and not for any dominant/nondominant comparison; this is consistent with the findings of Hollman et al. [28], who report no significant dominant/nondominant differences for a fractal exponent during knee extension or flexion constant-force tasks. Similar to this study, Hollman et al. [28] employed a mixed male/female sample. Different from this study, Hollman et al. [28] employed a mixed adult/adolescent sample and did not specify explicitly how the dominant limb was defined. Accordingly, because growth and development affect knee neuromuscular control [39] and limb dominance changes according to the nature of the task (e.g., load-bearing vs. skill) [10], the findings of Hollman et al. [28] are likely not comparable to the present study. Given that the present study identified a significant finding for a right/left comparison but not for a dominant/nondominant comparison, careful consideration should underpin the clinical reasoning for which a comparison method is employed because different statistical findings are evident for one method versus another; this is supported by the finding that side-to-side effect-sizes were substantially different between comparison methods for both ApEn and DFA α (Tables 2 and 3).

Previous research has analyzed side-to-side differences in variability, with equivocal results. Adam, Luca, and Erim [40] observed a significantly greater magnitude of variability in the nondominant first dorsal interosseous, whilst Bernardi et al. [41] observed no difference between dominant and nondominant limbs. The present study indicates potential side-to-side differences in the complexity of muscle output, with the left limb exhibiting lower complexity, as indicated by greater DFA α (Table 3). Moreover, there were no significant differences for either side-to-side comparison method for CV (Table 1). This supports the notion that complexity-based metrics may be more sensitive to subtle side-to-side differences than variability-based metrics [42]. It is, however, still recommended to use both magnitude- and complexity-based metrics for a thorough evaluation of signal fluctuations [17].

That there was a significant difference for the right/left DFA α comparison but not the right/left ApEn comparison supports the notion that these metrics assess subtly different aspects of complexity [21]. Because ApEn measures the regularity/randomness of a time series across one time scale [22], and DFA α measures fractal scaling across multiple time scales [21], agreement between the two metrics is not guaranteed. The insensitivity of one metric does not imply that other metrics will not yield meaningful information about a physiological system's functionality [43]. That side-to-side effect-size findings for right/left ApEn and DFA α are not similar (Tables 2 and 3) supports the notion that each variable provides unique information about knee extensor neuromuscular control complexity. Researchers should, therefore, use both ApEn and DFA α to assess knee neuromuscular control complexity, regardless of whether right/left or dominant/nondominant side-to-side comparisons are made.

Complex fluctuations in physiological signals represent the range across which biological systems operate and their ability to respond and adapt to stressors [16]. For both comparison methods, there was no significant side-to-side difference for ApEn (Table 2), suggesting that adaptability in knee extensor neuromuscular control is similar between sides. However, the medium-to-large effect size for the right/left ApEn comparison (Table 2) may indicate that side-to-side adaptability does actually differ. The significant side-to-side difference and very large effect size for the right/left DFA α (Table 3) supports the perspective that side-to-side adaptability in knee extensor neuromuscular control is different in uninjured individuals. Potential differences in the complexity of knee extensor neuromuscular control are reflective of differences in coordination and could have implications for the risk of injury [18]. Indeed, low complexity has been speculated to reflect a narrowing of system responsiveness and lower adaptability, which could increase the risk of failing a motor task and have a detrimental effect on functional movements [33].

Based on the coherence between the cumulative motor unit spike train (measured using high-density EMG) and muscle force output [44], variations in common synaptic input to the motor unit are the main determinant of the magnitude of force fluctuations [45]. Increased common synaptic input has also been speculated to be associated with lower complexity [33]. In support of the potential side-to-side differences in complexity, differences in motor unit synchronization (a necessary consequence of common synaptic input) have been observed between the muscles of the dominant/nondominant hand [40,46]. Such differences in motor unit discharge properties have, however, only been observed in the muscles of the hand, which may be subject to greater preferential use than the knee extensors during daily activities [47].

At the individual level, symmetry analyses examine whether clinically-significant side-to-side differences exist for an individual's mean or maximum values [13]. An absolute-asymmetry threshold of 15% was chosen because mean LSIs of approximately 85% are reported for isometric knee extension MVEs in uninjured individuals [34]. The mean absolute asymmetries for right/left and dominant/nondominant comparisons of CV and ApEn were >15% (Tables 4 and 5), whereas the mean absolute asymmetries for both comparisons for DFA α were $\leq$5% (Table 6). The magnitude of the mean absolute asymmetry was consistent regardless of whether a right/left or dominant/nondominant comparison was performed. Because the mean absolute asymmetry ranged from 4.9 to 34.5% across all variables and side-to-side comparison methods (Tables 4–6), further work is needed to determine whether the isometric knee extension strength mean LSIs of approximately 85% [34] and corresponding absolute asymmetries of 15% apply to variability and complexity measures.

The present study had some limitations. First, this study was a secondary analysis of a previously published work and was confined to a total sample size created from two separate primary studies [32,33]. Therefore, it was not possible to perform an *a priori* power analysis and our findings may include type 2 errors. Future primary research should ensure *a priori* power analyses are performed to facilitate adequate statistical power. Second, we did not undertake a *post hoc* power analysis. A *post hoc* power analysis uses the *p*-value returned from significance tests; given that nonsignificant *p*-values always correspond to low beta values and power, *post hoc* power analyses fail to add value to interpretations of research findings and are discouraged [48]. Again, future primary research should ensure that a priori power analyses are performed to reduce the risk of committing type 2 errors. Third, we were confined by the methods used in the original work, which only used one sub-maximal level of effort (50% MVE). Variability and complexity can vary with the level of isometric efforts [17]. Future primary studies should assess a variety of sub-maximal levels to reveal potential differences in knee neuromuscular control complexity. Fourth, limb dominance was defined by the preferred kicking limb rather than the strongest limb. Although it is possible that participants may have mistakenly and incorrectly self-reported one side as their dominant side, the subjectively reported preferred kicking limb is the method commonly employed in the literature for determining lower limb dominance [10]. Future research should compare different methods of defining and objectively determining limb dominance and how it affects the variability and complexity of side-to-side absolute asymmetries.

5. Conclusions

This is the first study to explore right/left and dominant/nondominant side-to-side comparisons of magnitude- and complexity-based metrics of knee neuromuscular control in uninjured individuals. A significant side-to-side difference and very large effect size existed for the right/left DFA α comparison, suggesting that side-to-side adaptability of knee extensor neuromuscular control in uninjured individuals is different. Side-to-side differences in the adaptability of knee extensor neuromuscular control may have clinical implications for the risk of future knee injury. Participants demonstrated a wide range of side-to-side absolute-asymmetries in knee neuromuscular control variability and complexity according to the comparison method used and the variable employed. Researchers should carefully consider which method is used for side-to-side comparisons and the threshold or range employed to define a clinically significant absolute asymmetry for each variable. Approximate entropy and DFA α assess subtly different aspects of complexity and both should be used alongside other traditional magnitude-based variables when studying knee neuromuscular control. The present analyses are practically significant because they provide new preliminary reference data that help to better understand the control of knee movement for both sides of the body and support the design of future larger-scale primary studies of motor control and knee health in uninjured and injured individuals.

Author Contributions: Conceptualization, N.C.C. and J.P.; methodology, N.C.C. and J.P.; formal analysis, N.C.C.; resources, J.P.; writing—original draft preparation, N.C.C. and J.P.; writing—review and editing, N.C.C. and J.P.; visualization, N.C.C. and J.P.; supervision, N.C.C.; project administration, N.C.C. All authors have read and agreed to the published version of the manuscript.

Funding: This research received no external funding.

Institutional Review Board Statement: This study was a secondary analysis of data collected for a larger primary research project. Ethics approval was obtained for the original primary research project.

Informed Consent Statement: This study was a secondary analysis of data collected for a larger primary research project. Informed consent was provided by all participants for the original primary research project.

Data Availability Statement: Because this study was a secondary analysis, no new data were created or analyzed in this study. Data sharing is not applicable to this article.

Conflicts of Interest: The authors declare no conflict of interest.

References

1. Kennedy, M.; Dunne, C.; Mulcahy, B.; Molloy, M. The sports clinic: A one year review of new referrals. *Ir. Med. J.* **1993**, *86*, 29–30. [PubMed]
2. Sarimo, J.; Rantanen, J.; Heikkilä, J.; Helttula, I.; Hiltunen, A.; Orava, S. Acute traumatic hemarthrosis of the knee. Is routine arthroscopic examination necessary? A study of 320 consecutive patients. *Scand. J. Surg.* **2002**, *91*, 361–364. [CrossRef] [PubMed]
3. Finch, C.; Cassell, E. The public health impact of injury during sport and active recreation. *J. Sci. Med. Sport* **2006**, *9*, 490–497. [CrossRef] [PubMed]
4. Lubowitz, J.H.; Appleby, D. Cost-Effectiveness Analysis of the Most Common Orthopaedic Surgery Procedures: Knee Arthroscopy and Knee Anterior Cruciate Ligament Reconstruction. *Arthroscopy* **2011**, *27*, 1317–1322. [CrossRef] [PubMed]
5. Lohmander, L.; Englund, P.; Dahl, L.; Roos, E. The Long-term Consequence of Anterior Cruciate Ligament and Meniscus Injuries: Osteoarthritis. *Am. J. Sports Med.* **2007**, *35*, 1756–1769. [CrossRef]
6. Avery, J. Accident prevention-injury control-injury prevention-or whatever? *Inj. Prev.* **1995**, *1*, 10–11. [CrossRef] [PubMed]
7. Clark, N.C. Functional performance testing following knee ligament injury. *Phys. Ther. Sport* **2001**, *2*, 91–105. [CrossRef]
8. Clark, N.C. Noncontact knee ligament injury prevention screening in netball: A clinical commentary with clinical practice suggestions for community-level players. *Int. J. Sports Phys. Ther.* **2021**, *16*, 911–929. [CrossRef]
9. Newton, R.; Gerber, A.; Nimphius, S.; Shim, J.; Doan, B.; Robertson, M.; Pearson, D.; Craig, B.; Häkkinen, K.; Kraemer, W. Determination of functional strength imbalance of the lower extremities. *J. Strength Cond. Res.* **2006**, *20*, 971–977.
10. McGrath, T.; Waddington, G.; Scarvell, J.; Ball, N.; Creer, R.; Woods, K.; Smith, D. The effect of limb dominance on lower limb functional performance—A systematic review. *J. Sports Sci.* **2016**, *34*, 289–302. [CrossRef]
11. Magee, D. *Orthopedic Physical Assessment*, 6th ed.; Elsevier: St. Louis, MO, USA, 2014.
12. Portney, L.; Watkins, M. *Foundations of Clinical Research: Applications to Practice*, 3rd ed.; Pearson/Prentice Hall: Upper Saddle River, NJ, USA, 2009.
13. Clark, N.C.; Mullally, E.M. Prevalence and magnitude of preseason clinically-significant single-leg balance and hop test asymmetries in an English adult netball club. *Phys. Ther. Sport* **2019**, *40*, 44–52. [CrossRef] [PubMed]
14. Clark, N.C.; Clacher, L.H. Lower-limb motor-performance asymmetries in English community-level female field hockey players: Implications for knee and ankle injury prevention. *Phys. Ther. Sport* **2020**, *43*, 43–51. [CrossRef] [PubMed]
15. Riemann, B.; Lephart, S. The sensorimotor system, part I: The physiologic basis of functional joint stability. *J. Athl. Train.* **2002**, *37*, 71–79. [PubMed]
16. Lipsitz, L.; Goldberger, A. Loss of 'complexity' and aging. Potential applications of fractals and chaos theory to senescence. *J. Am. Med. Assoc.* **1992**, *267*, 1806–1809. [CrossRef]

17. Slifkin, A.B.; Newell, K.M. Noise, information transmission, and force variability. *J. Exp. Psychol.* **1999**, *25*, 837–851. [CrossRef]
18. Stergiou, N.; Decker, L.M. Human movement variability, nonlinear dynamics, and pathology: Is there a connection? *Hum. Mov. Sci.* **2011**, *30*, 869–888. [CrossRef]
19. Enoka, R.M.; Christou, E.A.; Hunter, S.K.; Kornatz, K.W.; Semmler, J.G.; Taylor, A.M.; Tracy, B.L. Mechanisms that contribute to differences in motor performance between young and old adults. *J. Electromyogr. Kinesiol.* **2003**, *13*, 1–12. [CrossRef]
20. Pethick, J.; Winter, S.L.; Burnley, M. Fatigue reduces the complexity of knee extensor torque fluctuations during maximal and submaximal intermittent isometric contractions in man. *J. Physiol.* **2015**, *593*, 2085–2096. [CrossRef]
21. Goldberger, A.L.; Amaral, L.A.; Hausdorff, J.M.; Ivanov, P.C.; Peng, C.-K.; Stanley, H.E. Fractal dynamics in physiology: Alterations with disease and aging. *Proc. Natl. Acad. Sci. USA* **2002**, *99*, 2466–2472. [CrossRef]
22. Pincus, S.M. Approximate entropy as a measure of system complexity. *Proc. Natl. Acad. Sci. USA* **1991**, *88*, 2297–2301. [CrossRef]
23. Paraschiv-Ionescu, A.; Buchser, E.; Rutschmann, B.; Aminian, K. Nonlinear analysis of human physical activity patterns in health and disease. *Phys. Rev. E* **2008**, *77*, 021913. [CrossRef] [PubMed]
24. Tigrini, A.; Verdini, F.; Fioretti, S.; Mengarelli, A. Long term correlation and inhomogeneity of the inverted pendulum sway time-series under the intermittent control paradigm. *Commun. Nonlinear Sci. Numer. Simul.* **2022**, *108*, 106198. [CrossRef]
25. Marmelat, V.; Meidinger, R.L. Fractal analysis of gait in people with Parkinson's disease: Three minutes is not enough. *Gait Posture* **2019**, *70*, 229–234. [CrossRef] [PubMed]
26. Vaillancourt, D.; Newell, K. Aging and the time and frequency structure of force output variability. *J. Appl. Physiol.* **2003**, *94*, 903–912. [CrossRef]
27. Goetschius, J.; Hart, J.M. Knee-extension torque variability and subjective knee function in patients with a history of anterior cruciate ligament reconstruction. *J. Athl. Train.* **2016**, *51*, 22–27. [CrossRef]
28. Hollman, J.H.; Nagai, T.; Bates, N.A.; McPherson, A.L.; Schilaty, N.D. Diminished neuromuscular system adaptability following anterior cruciate ligament injury: Examination of knee muscle force variability and complexity. *Clin. Biomech.* **2021**, *90*, 105513. [CrossRef]
29. Gibson, F.; Fern, L.A.; Phillips, B.; Gravestock, H.; Malik, S.; Callaghan, A.; Dyker, K.; Groszmann, M.; Hamrang, L.; Hough, R. Reporting the whole story: Analysis of the 'out-of-scope'questions from the James Lind Alliance Teenage and Young Adult Cancer Priority Setting Partnership Survey. *Health Expect.* **2021**, *24*, 1593–1606. [CrossRef]
30. Boslaugh, S. *Secondary Data Sources for Public Health. A Practical Guide*; Cambridge University Press: Cambridge, UK, 2007.
31. Lewis-Beck, M.; Bryaman, A.; Liao, T. *Secondary Analysis of Quantitative Data—The SAGE Encyclopedia of Social Science Research Methods*; Sage Publications: Thousand Oaks, CA, USA, 2004.
32. Pethick, J.; Winter, S.L.; Burnley, M. Effects of ipsilateral and contralateral fatigue and muscle blood flow occlusion on the complexity of knee-extensor torque output in humans. *Exp. Physiol.* **2018**, *103*, 956–967. [CrossRef]
33. Pethick, J.; Whiteaway, K.; Winter, S.L.; Burnley, M. Prolonged depression of knee-extensor torque complexity following eccentric exercise. *Exp. Physiol.* **2019**, *104*, 100–111. [CrossRef]
34. Lisee, C.; Slater, L.; Hertel, J.; Hart, J.M. Effect of sex and level of activity on lower-extremity strength, functional performance, and limb symmetry. *J. Sport Rehabil.* **2019**, *28*, 413–420. [CrossRef]
35. Peng, C.-K.; Buldyrev, S.V.; Havlin, S.; Simons, M.; Stanley, H.E.; Goldberger, A.L. Mosaic organization of DNA nucleotides. *Phys. Rev. E* **1994**, *49*, 1685–1689. [CrossRef] [PubMed]
36. Richman, J.S.; Moorman, J.R. Physiological time-series analysis using approximate entropy and sample entropy. *Am. J. Physiol.-Heart Circ. Physiol.* **2000**, *278*, H2039–H2049. [CrossRef] [PubMed]
37. Forrest, S.M.; Challis, J.H.; Winter, S.L. The effect of signal acquisition and processing choices on ApEn values: Towards a "gold standard" for distinguishing effort levels from isometric force records. *Med. Eng. Phys.* **2014**, *36*, 676–683. [CrossRef] [PubMed]
38. Pethick, J.; Winter, S.L.; Burnley, M. Relationship between muscle metabolic rate and muscle torque complexity during fatiguing intermittent isometric contractions in humans. *Physiol. Rep.* **2019**, *7*, e14240. [CrossRef]
39. DiStefano, L.; Martinez, J.; Crowley, E.; Matteau, E.; Kerner, M.; Boling, M.; Nguyen, A.; Trojian, T. Maturation and sex differences in neuromuscular characteristics of youth athletes. *J. Strength Cond. Res.* **2015**, *29*, 2465–2473. [CrossRef]
40. Adam, A.; Luca, C.J.D.; Erim, Z. Hand dominance and motor unit firing behavior. *J. Neurophysiol.* **1998**, *80*, 1373–1382. [CrossRef]
41. Bernardi, M.; Felici, F.; Marchetti, M.; Montellanico, F.; Piacentini, M.; Solomonow, M. Force generation performance and motor unit recruitment strategy in muscles of contralateral limbs. *J. Electromyogr. Kinesiol.* **1999**, *9*, 121–130. [CrossRef]
42. Vaillancourt, D.; Slifkin, A.; Newell, K. Regularity of force tremor in Parkinson's disease. *Clin. Neurophysiol.* **2001**, *112*, 1594–1603. [CrossRef]
43. Pethick, J.; Winter, S.L.; Burnley, M. Fatigue reduces the complexity of knee extensor torque during fatiguing sustained isometric contractions. *Eur. J. Sport Sci.* **2019**, *19*, 1349–1358. [CrossRef]
44. Negro, F.; Holobar, A.; Farina, D. Fluctuations in isometric muscle force can be described by one linear projection of low-frequency components of motor unit discharge rates. *J. Physiol.* **2009**, *587*, 5925–5938. [CrossRef]
45. Farina, D.; Negro, F. Common synaptic input to motor neurons, motor unit synchronization, and force control. *Exerc. Sport Sci. Rev.* **2015**, *43*, 23–33. [CrossRef] [PubMed]
46. Schmied, A.; Vedel, J.-P.; Pagni, S. Human spinal lateralization assessed from motoneurone synchronization: Dependence on handedness and motor unit type. *J. Physiol.* **1994**, *480*, 369–387. [CrossRef] [PubMed]

47. Williams, D.; Sharma, S.; Bilodeau, M. Neuromuscular fatigue of elbow flexor muscles of dominant and non-dominant arms in healthy humans. *J. Electromyogr. Kinesiol.* **2002**, *12*, 287–294. [CrossRef]
48. Hoenig, J.M.; Heisey, D.M. The abuse of power: The pervasive fallacy of power calculations for data analysis. *Am. Stat.* **2001**, *55*, 19–24. [CrossRef]

 applied sciences

MDPI

Article

Changes in Spinal-Reflex Excitability during Static Stretch and/or Explosive Contraction

Kyeong Eun Min [1], YongSuk Lee [2] and Jihong Park [3,*]

[1] Athletic Training Laboratory, Department of Physical Education, Graduate School, Kyung Hee University, Yongin 17104, Korea; mke92@khu.ac.kr
[2] Athletic Training Laboratory, Department of Sports Medicine and Science, Graduate School of Physical Education, Kyung Hee University, Yongin 17104, Korea; donkey00@khu.ac.kr
[3] Athletic Training Laboratory, Department of Sports Medicine, Kyung Hee University, Yongin 17104, Korea
* Correspondence: jihong.park@khu.ac.kr; Tel.: +82-31-201-2721

Abstract: To examine individual or combined effects of static stretch and explosive contraction on quadriceps spinal-reflex excitability (the peak Hoffmann's reflex normalized by the peak motor-response) and the latency times of the Hoffmann's reflex and motor-response. Fourteen healthy young males randomly experienced four conditions (stretch, contraction, stretch + contraction, and control—no intervention). For the stretch condition, three sets of a 30 s hold using the modified Thomas test on each leg were performed. For the contraction condition, three trials of maximal countermovement vertical jump were performed. Quadriceps spinal-reflex excitability and the latent period of each value on the right leg were compared at pre- and post-condition. All measurement values across conditions were not changed at any time point (condition × time) in spinal-reflex excitability ($F_{6,143} = 1.10$, $p = 0.36$), Hoffmann's reflex latency ($F_{6,143} = 0.45$, $p = 0.84$), motor-response latency ($F_{6,143} = 0.37$, $p = 0.90$), and vertical jump heights ($F_{2,65} = 1.82$, $p = 0.17$). A statistical trend was observed in the contraction condition that spinal-reflex excitability was increased by 42% (effect size: 0.63). Neither static stretch nor explosive contraction changed the quadriceps spinal-reflex excitability, latency of Hoffmann's reflex, and motor-response. Since our stretch protocol did not affect jumping performance and our contraction protocol induced the post-activation potentiation effect, either protocol could be used as pre-exercise activity.

Keywords: H:M ratio; Thomas test; vertical jump

Citation: Min, K.E.; Lee, Y.; Park, J. Changes in Spinal-Reflex Excitability during Static Stretch and/or Explosive Contraction. *Appl. Sci.* **2021**, *11*, 2830. https://doi.org/10.3390/app11062830

Academic Editor: Nyeonju Kang

Received: 2 March 2021
Accepted: 19 March 2021
Published: 22 March 2021

1. Introduction

Performance enhancement after warm-up activity could be explained by thermal and non-thermal effects. While the term "warm-up" is derived from the thermal effects due to any given activity (e.g., increased core body and local muscle temperatures), "pre-conditioning" [1], the working of muscles by performing sports movements (e.g., explosive movements), is considered to contribute the non-thermal effects of warming-up [2]. Assuming the thermal effects are similar, the level of performance among different types of warm-up would be affected by the ability to utilize elastic energy [3]. Elastic energy is associated with muscle spindle activity [4], myotatic reflex [5], and elasticity of contractile components [6]. Measures of elastic energy are difficult because they are derived from various structures (e.g., actin, myosin, sarcolemma, tendon, etc.) that are instantiated through different neural pathways (e.g., α and γ motoneuron). Spinal-reflex excitability, Hoffmann (H)-reflex [7] normalized by the motor (M)-response (H:M ratio), is an autonomic homonymous response to a given peripheral (especially Ia afferent) stimulus [8]. Exogenous electrical stimuli should directly evoke afferents; the H-reflex bypasses the signals of muscle spindles and γ-motoneurons [9]. It has been suggested that the magnitude of the stretch-reflex is related to the amount of stored elastic energy [10,11]. The amplitude of this value is indicative of synaptic transmission [2], spinally mediated neural inhibition [12], and an estimate of α-motoneuron activity [13]. Additionally, the assessment of the H-reflex and M-response latency time are also considered to be parameters affecting synaptic transmission along with performance change [14]. Therefore, the non-thermal effects of warming-up in terms of enhancing elastic potential energy could be assessed by spinal-reflex excitability and the latency times of the H-reflex and the M-response.

Previous studies concerning the acute change in the soleus H-reflex reported a reduction after static stretch [15,16] and an increase after muscle contractions [17,18]. Although the existing data inform us how the H-reflex responds to stretch or contraction, several limitations still need to be addressed. First, spinal-reflex excitability in the quadriceps has not been examined even though it is the primary muscle for functional movements [19,20]. Second, subjects in previous reports examined isometric contractions [17,18], which are not commonly performed during warming-up or training. Third, the combined effect of stretch and contraction is unknown. For example, reduced spinal-reflex excitability after performing static stretch might be offset by performing muscle contractions such as maximal vertical jumps. This indicates that static stretch does not produce performance hinderance if vertical jumps are followed. Knowing the direction and magnitude of change in spinally mediated muscle activation of quadriceps responding to static stretch and/or explosive contraction would help coaches and athletes to plan and execute pre-exercise activities. While the general hesitance of static stretch to hamper muscle power in the field of exercise science still exists, comparing jump heights before and after static stretch would also provide a comprehensive understanding of the relationships among static stretch, quadriceps spinal-reflex excitability, and athletic performance.

A comparison of the individual and combined effects of static stretch (e.g., hip and knee extensors) and explosive contraction (e.g., maximal vertical jump) could address the limitations above, and thus provide information on the relationship between spinal-reflex excitability and athletic performance as well as the interaction effect between muscle stretch and contraction. Therefore, the purpose of this study was to examine the immediate effects of static stretch and/or two-legged maximal vertical jump on quadriceps spinal-reflex excitability, and the latency time of the H-reflex and M-response, compared with no activity which served as the control. Based on previous reports on the soleus H-reflex [15–18], it can be hypothesized that quadriceps spinal-reflex excitability would be decreased after stretching and increased after contracting (jumping). Since change in quadriceps spinal-reflex excitability after stretch or contraction is unknown, it is difficult to predict the result of the combined condition (stretch and contraction). If the magnitudes of change after stretch or contraction were similar, the effects of two stimuli would be cancelled out, resulting in no change. While change in the latency time can be indicative of temporal change in neural activation, a previous study [21] reported that static stretch or vibration did not change the H-reflex and M-response latency time in the soleus. According to that, we hypothesized no change in the H-reflex and M-response latency time across the four conditions.

2. Materials and Methods

2.1. Subjecs

We recruited recreationally active male individuals (aged between 19 and 25; exercise > 3 times a week at moderate intensity; a total exercise duration between 150 min and 250 min for the last six months) who had a measurable quadriceps (vastus medialis: VM) H-reflex and M-response. Subjects had no history of lower-back or -body surgery and were free from lower-back or -body injuries in the past six months. Subjects with athletic career (experience of registration in the varsity team roaster or participation in an official sporting event) or cardiovascular or neurological pathology were also excluded. Fifty-four subjects were initially screened, and 40 of them were excluded due to immeasurable H-reflex (n = 38) and unstable M-response (n = 2). Therefore, fourteen subjects (age: 23 ± 1 years; height: 175 ± 7 cm; mass: 69 ± 8 kg; exercise duration: 220 ± 79.4 min/week) were finally analyzed. Prior to participation, all subjects gave informed consent, approved by the university's Institutional Review Board, which also approved the study.

2.2. Testing Procedures

All subjects visited the laboratory four times on separate days at the same time of the day, 48 h apart. Subjects were asked to maintain their habitual diets during the experimental period and to refrain from any physical activity for 24 h prior to data collection. For the first session, subjects were screened for measurable H-reflex after providing informed consent. Ambient temperature and relative humidity within the laboratory were set as 25 °C and 50% during the data collection period. Upon arrival to the laboratory, subjects laid down on the treatment table and rested for 15 min to achieve spinal-reflex and cardiovascular stability prior to the screening. During this rest period, the VM on the dominant limb (i.e., the leg used to kick a ball) were shaved, debrided (with sandpaper), and cleaned with alcohol prep wipes before the placement of self-adhesive surface electromyography (EMG) electrodes (Ag-AgCI; EL 503-10; Biopac System Inc., Goleta, CA, USA). Two EMG electrodes (2 cm apart) were attached to the bulk of the VM. The ground electrode was attached to the medial malleolus of the ipsilateral limb.

During the H-reflex and M-response measurements, subjects were asked to place their hands along their sides with their palms kept supinated and to maintain this position as they looked at a spot on the ceiling while listening to white noise through earphones to avoid any possible sound-induced variability in measurements [22]. The stimulating module (Biopac STM 100C), isolation adaptor (Biopac Stimsoc), and a bar stimulation electrode (EL 503, Biopac Systems Inc., Goleta, CA, USA) provided the electrical stimulus over the femoral nerve (just lateral and/or down to the femoral artery). The peak H-reflex and peak M-response were found and recorded through surface EMG (sampling rate: 2000 Hz). Electrical stimulation was gradually increased at 0.1–2 V increments, with a 15 s rest between stimulations [23]. The average intensities (ranges) to elicit the peak H-reflex and the peak M-response were 6.0 (4.0 to 9.0) and 9.3 (7.1 to 10.0) V, respectively. Once peak amplitude was found, the same intensity was applied four times for the pre-condition measurements.

After the pre-condition measurements, the researcher who took measurements left, and the other researcher who was blinded to pre-condition measurements guided the intervention conditions in the laboratory. Subjects randomly experienced one of four conditions on each visit (stretch, contraction, stretch and contraction, and control: Figure 1). The order of the conditions for each subject was determined by the opaque envelope method. For the stretch condition, the modified Thomas test [24] was used. Subjects were asked to seat at the end of a treatment table and roll back onto the table while bending and pulling one of the knees to their chest. Once subjects were in the position, the researcher gradually provided manual stretch force (Figure 2). Subjects were asked to stop the researcher when they felt stretch sensation [25] or the point of discomfort [26], then this end position was held for 30 s, which was timed by the researcher. Three repetitions on each leg were alternatively performed (a total duration of 90 s with a rest interval of 30 s). For the contraction condition, subjects performed two-legged countermovement maximal vertical jumps on Vertec (Sports Imports, Hilliard, OH, USA). Subjects' standing arm reach height was measured with a Vertec. Subjects stood (same feet positions for vertical jumps) and maintained their lower-extremity full extension and trunk upright and raised (full scapular upward rotation with abduction) their dominant arm (i.e., the arm throwing a ball) directly overhead as high as possible. Subjects were then asked to vertically jump off of both legs as high as they possibly could and touch the plastic vane of the Vertec (this instruction was given during the standing arm height measurement). A self-selected pre-stretch of the lower-body and trunk and double-arm swinging at take-off were allowed. Three trials were performed, with a 30 s rest interval between jumps. For the stretch and contraction condition, the order of stretch and contraction interventions, described above, was performed. In the case of the conditions with contraction (contraction, and stretch and contraction), subjects performed a total of nine countermovement vertical jumps (condition: ×3; post-condition at 0 min; ×3; post-condition at 20 min: ×3; Figure 1). For the control condition, subjects neither performed stretching nor jumping but maintained a supine position on the treatment table. In this study, interventions (stretch and/or jump) were performed without specific warm-up activity to eliminate the potential confounding effects of change in tissue temperature or energy expenditure.

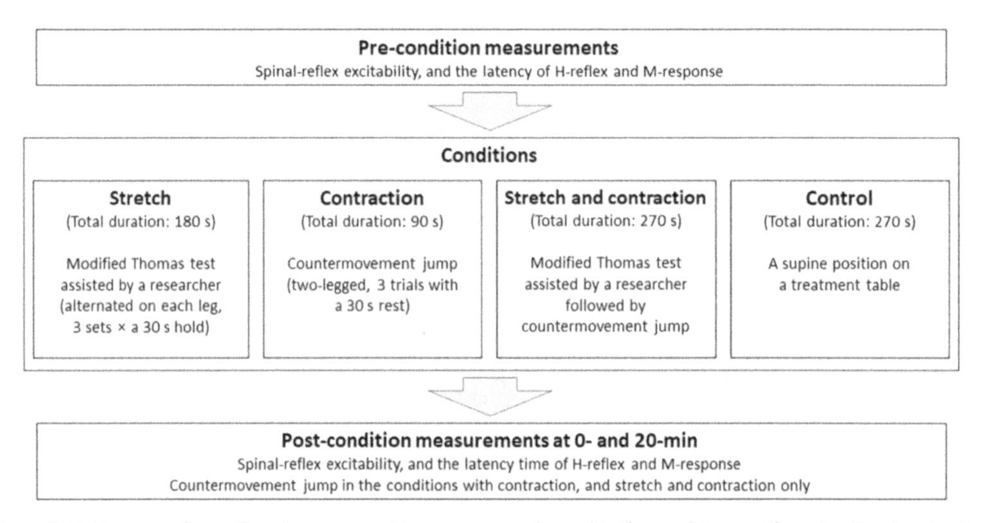

Figure 1. Testing procedures. Countermovement jumps were performed in the conditions with contraction (contraction, and stretch and contraction) during the conditions (×3), and post-condition at 0 (×3) and 20 min (×3).

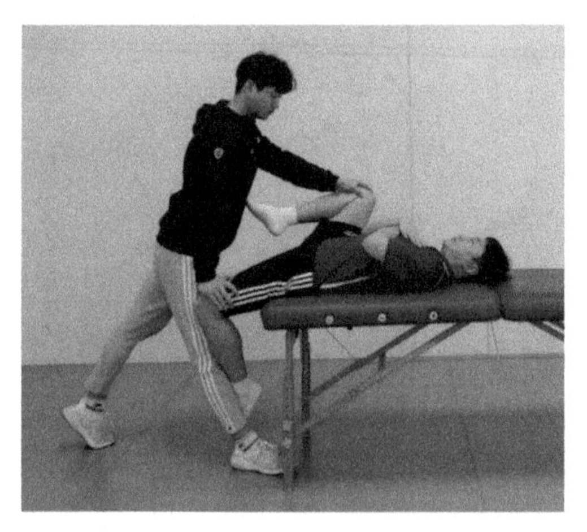

Figure 2. A subject performing stretch using the modified Thomas test. The researcher gradually provided an additional tensional force until the patient felt a self-selected moderate discomfort, then held the position for 30 s. The left hip flexors and right knee extensors are being stretched.

After the conditions, the researcher who guided the interventions left, and the other researcher who obtained measurements came into the laboratory. The post-condition measurements at 0 and 20 min were subsequently taken in the same manner as the pre-condition.

2.3. Data Reduction

The H:M ratio (the peak H-reflex normalized by the peak M-response) was calculated to obtain spinal-reflex excitability [27]. The latency times for the peak H-reflex and the peak M-response were also analyzed. Latent period was defined as the time between the stimulation onset and the peak H-reflex or the peak M-response [28]. Two-legged countermovement maximal vertical jump heights were calculated by subtracting the height of standing arm reach from the jump height. Jump height values were read in inches on Vertec then converted into centimeters.

2.4. Statistical Analysis

Our sample size was determined using an expected change in the H:M ratio of 0.12 and a standard deviation of 0.15, which yielded an effect size (ES) of 0.8 [29]. This estimation with an α of 0.05 and a β of 0.2 resulted in 13 individuals necessary in each condition.

To test condition effect over time, a mixed model analysis of variance (random variable: subjects; fixed variables: condition and time) was performed in the quadriceps spinal-reflex excitability and the latency of the H-reflex and M-response (4×3) and countermovement maximal vertical jump (2×3). Tukey–Kramer pairwise comparisons were performed for post-hoc tests ($p \leq 0.05$). To determine practical significance, between-time ES were also calculated [30]. To obtain measurement consistency on within- and between-session, two-way mixed model analysis of variance was performed using the pre-condition measurement values. Between-subject mean square and error mean square were then inserted into the formula to gain intraclass correlation coefficient (ICC) [31]. All data were analyzed using a statistical package SAS 9.4.

3. Results

3.1. Spinal-Reflex Excitability

We did not observe condition effect over time in quadriceps spinal-reflex excitability (condition × time: $F_{6,143} = 1.10$, $p = 0.36$; time effect: $F_{2,143} = 0.05$, $p = 0.95$; Table 1). Regardless of time (condition effect: $F_{3,143} = 2.39$, $p = 0.07$), statistical trends showed there was greater spinal-reflex excitability in the contraction condition than the stretch ($p = 0.03$, ES = 0.35, 19%) or stretch and contraction ($p = 0.05$, ES = 0.36, 18%) conditions (Figure 3). An additional statistical trend was observed (Figure 4) in the contraction condition such that spinal-reflex excitability increased (pre- vs. post-condition at 0 min: $p = 0.03$, ES = 0.63, 42%) and the increased value was sustained for 20 min (pre- vs. post-condition at 20 min: $p = 0.11$, ES = 0.46, 23%).

Table 1. Change in spinal-reflex excitability.

	Stretch	Contraction	Stretch and Contraction	Control
Pre-condition	0.24 (0.18 to 0.30)	0.22 (0.17 to 0.27)	0.24 (0.17 to 0.31)	0.26 (0.19 to 0.33)
Post-condition at 0 min	0.20 (0.14 to 0.26)	0.31 (0.22 to 0.40)	0.21 (0.13 to 0.29)	0.26 (0.20 to 0.32)
Post-condition at 20 min	0.22 (0.18 to 0.26)	0.28 (0.19 to 0.37)	0.22 (0.16 to 0.28)	0.26 (0.20 to 0.32)

The values are mean (lower and upper bounds of 95% confidence intervals).

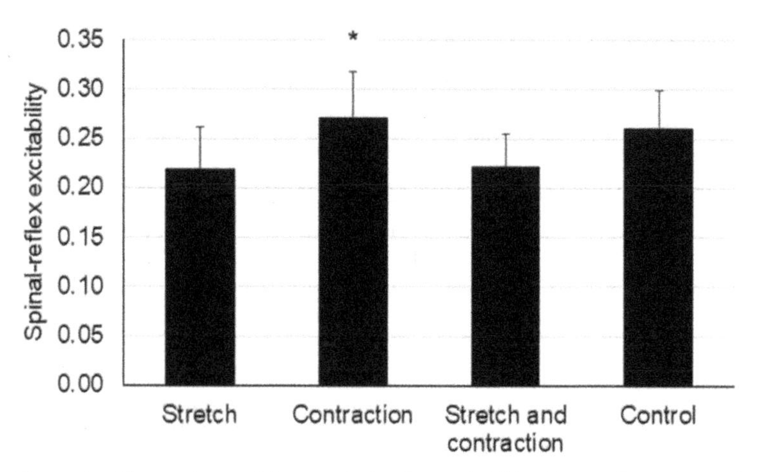

Figure 3. Change in quadriceps spinal-reflex excitability (time-collapsed: condition effect: $F_{3,143} = 2.39$, $p = 0.07$). * Different from the stretch condition ($p = 0.03$, ES = 0.35, 19%) and stretch and contraction condition ($p = 0.05$, ES = 0.36, 18%).

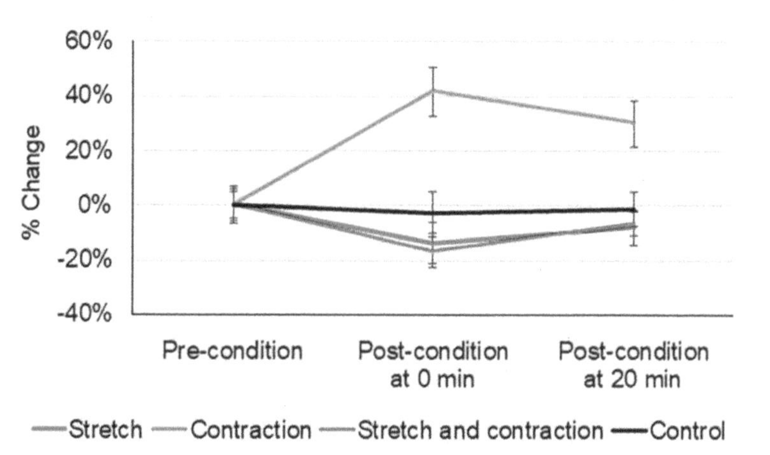

Figure 4. Quadriceps spinal-reflex excitability expressed as percentage change from the pre-condition measurement. Error bars are upper and lower values of 95% confidence intervals. After the contraction condition, quadriceps spinal-reflex excitability was increased at post-condition at 0 min (42%, ES = 0.63), and the increased value was maintained for 20 min (30%, ES = 0.46).

3.2. Latency of the H-Reflex and M-Response

The peak H-reflex latency (condition × time: $F_{6,143} = 0.45$, $p = 0.84$; condition effect: $F_{3,143} = 3.40$, $p = 0.02$; time effect: $F_{2,143} = 1.74$, $p = 0.18$; Table 2) and the peak M-response latency (condition × time: $F_{6,143} = 0.37$, $p = 0.90$; condition effect: $F_{3,143} = 1.30$, $p = 0.28$; time effect: $F_{2,143} = 1.20$, $p = 0.30$; Table 2) were analyzed.

Table 2. Change in the latency time.

	Peak H-Reflex (ms)				Peak M-Response (ms)			
	Stretch	Contraction	Stretch and Contraction	Control	Stretch	Contraction	Stretch and Contraction	Control
Pre-condition	17.2 (16.1 to 18.3)	17.6 (16.6 to 18.6)	17.4 (16.2 to 18.6)	16.3 (5.2 to 17.4)	6.3 (6.0 to 6.6)	6.3 (6.0 to 6.6)	6.1 (5.8 to 6.4)	6.1 (5.5 to 6.7)
Post-condition at 0 min	16.8 (15.4 to 18.2)	16.7 (15.6 to 17.8)	16.9 (15.6 to 18.2)	16.0 (14.9 to 17.1)	6.2 (5.9 to 6.5)	6.1 (5.8 to 6.4)	6.1 (5.8 to 6.4)	6.1 (5.5 to 6.7)
Post-condition at 20 min	16.0 (14.6 to 17.4)	17.0 (15.9 to 18.1)	17.2 (16.0 to 18.4)	16.1 (15.1 to 17.1)	6.4 (5.9 to 6.9)	6.2 (5.8 to 6.6)	6.4 (6.0 to 6.8)	6.1 (5.6 to 6.6)

The values are mean (lower and upper bounds of 95% confidence intervals).

3.3. *Two-Legged Maximal Countermovement Vertical Jump*

Two-legged countermovement maximal vertical jump heights did not differ between conditions at any time point (condition × time: $F_{2,65} = 1.82$, $p = 0.17$; time effect: $F_{2,65} = 0.21$, $p = 0.81$; Table 3). Regardless of time (condition effect: $F_{1,65} = 10.09$, $p = 0.002$), subjects in the stretch and contraction condition (49.8 cm) jumped higher than in the contraction condition (48.6 cm, ES = 0.12).

Table 3. Change in two-legged countermovement maximal vertical jump height.

Unit: cm	Contraction	Stretch and Contraction
Condition	48.4 (43.2 to 53.6)	50.1 (45.3 to 54.9)
Post-condition at 0 min	48.6 (43.4 to 53.8)	50.0 (45.1 to 54.9)
Post-condition at 20 min	49.0 (43.7 to 54.3)	49.1 (44.1 to 54.1)

The values are mean (lower and upper bounds of 95% confidence intervals). Note that the conditions with stretch and control did not perform maximal vertical jumps.

3.4. *Measurement Consistency*

Measurement consistency for each dependent variable at pre-condition was moderate to high (ICC values in spinal-reflex excitability: 0.85 to 0.99; H-reflex latency: 0.63 to 0.99; M-response latency: 0.77 to 0.99; and maximal countermovement vertical jump height: 0.93 to 0.97). All values including mean, standard deviation, and standard error of measurement (SEM) are presented in Table 4.

Table 4. Mean (SD), ICC, and SEM of spinal-reflex excitability, H-reflex and M-response latency time, and two-legged countermovement maximal vertical jump height at the pre-condition values.

Condition	Measurements	Mean (SD)	ICC	SEM
Stretch	Spinal-reflex excitability	0.24 (0.14)	0.99	0.01
	Peak H-reflex latency	17.18 (2.03)	0.99	0.20
	Peak M-response latency	6.29 (0.61)	0.99	0.06
Contraction	Spinal-reflex excitability	0.22 (0.10)	0.97	0.02
	Peak H-reflex latency	17.57 (1.91)	0.99	0.19
	Peak M-response latency	6.29 (0.61)	0.99	0.06
	Maximal vertical jump height	48.4 (10.0)	0.96	1.81
Stretch and contraction	Spinal-reflex excitability	0.24 (0.12)	0.99	0.01
	Peak H-reflex latency	17.36 (2.21)	0.99	0.21
	Peak M-response latency	6.07 (0.62)	0.99	0.06
	Maximal vertical jump height	50.1 (9.1)	0.97	1.83
Control	Spinal-reflex excitability	0.26 (0.14)	0.99	0.02
	Peak H-reflex latency	16.27 (2.10)	0.99	0.20
	Peak M-response latency	6.07 (0.62)	0.99	0.06

Table 4. *Cont.*

Condition	Measurements	Mean (SD)	ICC	SEM
Intersession	Spinal-reflex excitability	0.24 (0.12)	0.85	0.05
	Peak H-reflex latency	17.09 (2.07)	0.63	1.24
	Peak M-response latency	6.18 (0.61)	0.77	0.29
	Maximal vertical jump height	47.2 (10.5)	0.93	2.73

Unit: ms for latency of the H-reflex and M-response and cm for maximal vertical jump height. Note that the stretch and control condition did not perform vertical jump. SD: standard deviation; ICC: intraclass correlation coefficient; SEM: standard error of measurement.

4. Discussion

The primary objective of our study was to observe immediate changes in quadriceps (VM) spinal-reflex excitability in response to static stretch and/or explosive contraction. The spinal-reflex excitability remained unchanged across conditions (stretch, contraction, stretch and contraction, control) by time (pre- to post-condition). However, our hypotheses that the quadriceps spinal-reflex excitability would be reduced by stretch or increased by contraction were partially supported by trends in the condition effect (time-collapsed, $p = 0.07$: Figure 3). Based on the results of the condition effect, static stretch seemed to attenuate the spinal-reflex excitability when combined with explosive contraction or not. Statistical trends (Figure 4) in each condition over time also support the hypothesized direction of change. However, small to moderate ESs (0.35 to 0.63) indicate that these spinal-reflex excitability changes in responding to static stretch and/or explosive contraction are small. As expected, the latency time in H-reflex and M-response did not change among conditions over time. According to many other studies [21,32], this observation suggests that muscle stretch or contraction does not alter the latency time.

4.1. Static Stretch and Jumping Performance

Although a large body of research [33–35] has shown decreases in athletic performance such as vertical jump, static stretch is still considered as a part of warm-up routines due to gains of tissue compliance [36], potential injury reduction [37], and performance enhancement [38]. Therefore, the practical importance of static stretch on countermovement vertical jump heights was tested as the secondary aim. Our stretch protocol volume (3 sets × 30 s hold, alternated on each leg) did not change jumping performance, which is in line with the study in which the same stretch volume was administered [39,40]. Overall jump heights (statistical condition effect) between the condition of contraction (48.6 cm) and stretch and contraction (49.8 cm) were different, but it is not a meaningful observation since the amount of difference was within the SEM (2.73 cm) and a small ES (0.12). Previously, a 60 s [41] or 90 s [42] hold static stretch on lower extremity led to a reduction in maximal vertical jump. Taken together, the use of intermittent static stretch may have a minimal or no detrimental effect on subsequent explosive performance, although the total duration of static stretch (90 s) exceeded the previously suggested threshold duration (> 60 s) [43,44]. Since nether the spinal-reflex excitability nor vertical jump heights show statistical changes, we do not know how the spinal-reflex excitability influenced vertical jump height. With scientific evidence on muscle spindle activation and α-motoneuron facilitation [45], our observation could be interpreted in a couple of ways: (1) Regardless of the magnitude, changed spinal-reflex excitability has a minimal effect on jumping performance; or (2) altered spinal-reflex excitability in this study was small, which was insufficient to affect explosive contraction. Examining spinal-reflex excitability along with other explanatory factors that include biomechanical and physiological variables during altered jump height after static stretch would provide better understanding of the causal relationship and mechanisms that affect jump height after static stretch.

4.2. Quadriceps Spinal-Reflex Excitability after Static Stretch and/or Explosive Contraction

Our study was the first attempt to observe changes in quadriceps spinal-reflex excitability in responding to static stretch and/or explosive contraction. The H-reflex is a monosynaptic response that is modulated by the magnitude of Ia sensory input and the sensitivity of muscle spindle activity [46]. The endings of muscle spindles respond to change in muscle length (e.g., speed and size) such as a quick muscle stretch or artificial electrical stimulation [47]. Stimulation of Golgi tendon organ after a certain period of static stretch (e.g., >6 s) overrides the impulses from the muscle spindles [48]. A decreased H-reflex after static stretch (e.g., via autogenic inhibition), therefore, could be interpreted as an inhibition of muscle spindle activity. This could be further indicative of a reduction in muscle activation and force development due to the innervation of α-γ coactivation system to muscle spindles [46]. Our hypotheses were based on previous studies that reported changes in the soleus H-reflex after static stretch [15,16] and isometric contraction [17,18]. We, however, did not observe such change (e.g., a statistical interaction on condition by time) in terms of quadriceps spinal-reflex excitability. We are unsure if changes in quadriceps spinal-reflex excitability are dose-dependent, and the volume of our stretch or contraction protocol did not reach the threshold point when excitability begins to alter significantly from baseline. Future studies should attempt to find this threshold, in terms of the volume and intensity, on quadriceps spinal-reflex excitability.

4.3. Statistical Trends and the Combined Effect

We observed there was a 14% reduction (ES = 0.27) after static stretch and a 42% increase (ES = 0.63) after explosive contraction in the spinal-reflex excitability. Although moderate, the calculated ES after vertical jumps (contraction condition) supports the general idea that muscle contractions (preconditioning) acutely produce the post-activation potentiation (PAP) effect, especially on spinal-level excitability [49,50]. Considering the importance of VM activation during functional movements [51,52], the facilitative effect after explosive contraction also has the practical implication that a countermovement vertical jump is an appropriate pre-exercise activity. We speculate that the increased spinal-reflex excitability in our study was attributed to acute adjustment in neural adaptation due to the Ia presynaptic inhibition [53] and/or motor unit recruitment [54]. The increased spinal-reflex excitability seen in our study gradually decreased toward baseline after a 20 min measurement interval between the post-condition at 0 and 20 min (Figure 4); this prolonged increase has been reported in previous studies [55,56]. Along with no change in vertical jump heights, our observation of spinal-reflex excitability suggests that factors, other than neural activation (e.g., contractile response, temperature change), must play a role in performance enhancement as a PAP stimulus [54]. The Ia spinal-reflex more likely responds to low-intensity contractions [57], which also partly explains why our results did not show statistical differences. An antagonistic effect was expected in the combined condition (stretch and contraction). However, the percent change in spinal-reflex excitability (a 17% reduction) in this condition was similar to that in the isolated stretch condition, suggesting that the tensional stimulus dampens the contraction stimulus.

4.4. Limitations and Assumptions

Training level is one of the contributing factors to the effects of static stretch on athletic performance [58]. Therefore, our subjects were not athletes but recreationally active such that their training background (e.g., experience and frequency of static stretch) must be acknowledged. Additionally, our results for the combined condition were based on three trials of vertical jumps. Typically, a larger volume of dynamic movements as pre-exercise activity are performed; hence, care should be taken not to over-generalize our results. Regarding the spinal-reflex excitability, it should be assumed that each subject's response and adaptation to the stimulus of static stretch were similar across sessions. While a pre-exercise activity including static stretch is performed at every practice (or on a regular basis), we do not know the level of response adaptation due to repetitive stimulation by static stretch on jumping performance. Lastly, we calculated the H:M ratio (recorded via the electrodes attached to the VM) to examine the quadriceps spinal-reflex excitability as many previous studies did [22,29,59,60]. The H-reflex and M-response were elicited by electrical stimulations to the femoral nerve, which innervates the entire quadriceps muscles. Therefore, we assume that the VM activation was not different to other quadriceps muscles.

4.5. Practical Implications

We observed that a 90 s hold lower quarter static stretch, either alone or in conjunction with vertical jumps, did not alter maximal jumping ability of recreationally active subjects. The observed level of jumping performance after either condition above (static stretch or static stretch followed by vertical jumps) was similar to that after the condition using sport-specific movement (vertical jumps). This also suggests that the isolated or combined effects of our protocols of the static stretch and explosive contraction could be incorporated into a warm-up activity.

5. Conclusions

Neither static stretch (in a modified Thomas test using a 30 s hold ×3 on each leg) nor explosive contraction (using two-legged maximal countermovement vertical jumps ×3) changed the quadriceps spinal-reflex excitability, and the latency time of the H-reflex and M-response. Since our stretch protocol did not affect jumping performance and our contraction protocol induced the PAP effect (increased the quadriceps spinal-reflex excitability by 42% with an ES of 0.63), either protocol could be used as a pre-exercise activity.

Author Contributions: Conceptualization, K.E.M. and J.P.; methodology, K.E.M., Y.L., J.P.; software, K.E.M. and Y.L.; formal analysis, K.E.M.; investigation, J.P.; resources, J.P.; data curation, K.E.M. and Y.L.; writing—original draft preparation, K.E.M. and J.P.; writing—review and editing, K.E.M. and J.P.; visualization, K.E.M. and J.P.; supervision, J.P.; project administration, J.P. All authors have read and agreed to the published version of the manuscript.

Funding: This work was supported by the IOC Research Centre KOREA, Wonju, Korea.

Institutional Review Board Statement: The study was conducted according to the guidelines of the Declaration of Helsinki and approved by the Institutional Review Board of Kyung Hee University (KHSIRB 2016-010).

Informed Consent Statement: Informed consent was obtained from all subjects involved in the study.

Data Availability Statement: The data are available on request from the corresponding author.

Conflicts of Interest: The authors declare no conflict of interest.

References

1. Safran, M.R.; Garrett, W.E., Jr.; Seaber, A.V.; Glisson, R.R.; Ribbeck, B.M. The role of warmup in muscular injury pervention. *Am. J. Sports Med.* **1988**, *16*, 123–129. [CrossRef]
2. Racinais, S.; Cocking, S.; Périard, J.D. Sports and environmental temperature: From warming-up to heating-up. *Temperature* **2017**, *40*, 227–257. [CrossRef]
3. Bobbert, M.F.; Gerritsen, K.G.; Litjens, M.C.; Van Soest, A.J. Why is countermovement jump height greater than squat jump height? *Med. Sci. Sports Exerc.* **1996**, *28*, 1402–1412. [CrossRef] [PubMed]
4. Fletcher, I.M.; Monte-Colombo, M.M. An investigation into the possible physiological mechanisms associated with changes in performance related to acute responses to different preactivity stretch modalities. *Appl. Physiol. Nut. Metabol.* **2010**, *35*, 27–34. [CrossRef]
5. Behm, D.G.; Chaouachi, A. A review of the acute effects of static and dynamic stretching on performance. *Eur. J. Appl. Physiol.* **2011**, *111*, 2633–2651. [CrossRef] [PubMed]
6. Horita, T.; Komi, P.; Nicol, C.; Kyröläinen, H. Stretch shortening cycle fatigue: Interactions among joint stiness, reflex, and muscle mechanical performance in the drop jump. *Eur. J. Appl. Physiol. Occup. Physiol.* **1996**, *73*, 393–403. [CrossRef] [PubMed]
7. Hoffman, P. Beitrag zur kenntnis der menschlichen reflexe mit besonderer berucksichtigung der elektrischen erscheinungen. *Arch. Anat. Physiol.* **1910**, *1*, 223–246.

8. Zehr, P.E. Considerations for use of the Hoffmann reflex in exercise studies. *Eur. J. Appl. Physiol.* **2002**, *86*, 455–468. [CrossRef]
9. Knikow, M. The H-reflex as a probe: Pathways and pitfalls. *J. Neurosci. Methods* **2008**, *171*, 1–12. [CrossRef]
10. Avela, J.; Komi, P.V. Reduced stretch reflex sensitivity and muscle stiffness after long-lasting stretch-shortening cycle exercise in humans. *Eur. J. Appl. Physiol.* **1998**, *78*, 403–410. [CrossRef]
11. Komi, P.V.; Gollhofer, A. Stretch reflexes can have an important role in force enhancement during ssc exercise. *J. Appl. Biomech.* **1997**, *13*, 451–460. [CrossRef]
12. Grindstaff, T.L.; Pietrosimone, B.G.; Sauer, L.D.; Kerringan, D.C.; Patrie, J.T.; Hertel, J.; Ingersoll, C.D. Manual therapy directed at the knee or lumbopelvic region does not influence quadriceps spinal-reflex excitability. *Man. Ther.* **2014**, *19*, 299–305. [CrossRef] [PubMed]
13. Hopkins, J.T.; Ingersoll, C.D.; Krause, B.A.; Edwards, J.E.; Cordova, M.L. Effect of knee joint effusion on quadriceps and soleus motoneuron pool excitability. *Med. Sci. Sports Exerc.* **2001**, *33*, 123–126. [CrossRef]
14. Ritzmann, R.; Kramer, A.; Gollhofer, A.; Taube, W. The effect of whole body vibration on the H-reflex, the stretch reflex, and the short-latency response during hopping. *Scand. J. Med. Sci. Sports* **2013**, *23*, 331–339. [CrossRef]
15. Nielsen, J.; Petersen, N.; Ballegaard, M.; Biering-Sørensen, F.; Kiehn, O. H-reflexes are less depressed following muscle stretch in spastic spinal cord injured patients than in healthy subjects. *Exp. Brain Res.* **1993**, *97*, 173–176. [CrossRef]
16. Avela, J.; Kyröläinen, H.; Komi, P.V. Altered reflex sensitivity after repeated and prolonged passive muscle stretching. *J. Appl. Physiol.* **1999**, *86*, 1283–1291. [CrossRef]
17. Hwang, I.S.; Huang, C.Y.; Wu, P.S.; Chen, W.C.; Wang, C.H. Assessment of H reflex sensitivity with M wave alteration consequent to fatiguing contractions. *Int. J. Neurosci.* **2008**, *118*, 1317–1330. [CrossRef]
18. Stuzig, N.; Siebert, T. Assessment of the H-reflex at two contraction levels before and after fatigue. *Scand. J. Med. Sci. Sports* **2017**, *27*, 399–407. [CrossRef] [PubMed]
19. Mizner, R.L.; Snyder-Mackler, L. Altered loading during walking and sit-to-stand is affected by quadriceps weakness after total knee arthroplasty. *J. Orthop. Res.* **2005**, *23*, 1083–1090. [CrossRef]
20. Keays, S.L.; Bullock-Saxton, J.; Newcombe, P.A.; Keays, A.C. The relationship between knee strength and functional stability before and after anterior cruciate ligament reconstruction. *J. Orthop. Res.* **2003**, *21*, 231–237. [CrossRef]
21. Yapicioglu, B.; Colakoglu, M.; Colakoglu, Z.; Gulluoglu, H.; Bademkiran, F.; Ozkaya, O. Effects of a dynamic warm-up, static stretching or static stretching with tendon vibration on vertical jump performance and EMG responses. *J. Hum. Kinet.* **2013**, *39*, 49–57. [CrossRef] [PubMed]
22. Park, J.; Hopkins, J.T. Immediate effects of acupuncture and cryotherapy on quadriceps motoneuron pool excitability: Randomised trial using anterior knee infusion model. *Acupuncrt. Med.* **2012**, *30*, 195–202. [CrossRef] [PubMed]
23. Kolosova, E.V.; Slivko, É.I. Fatigue-induced modulation of the H reflex of soleus muscle in humans. *Neurophysiology* **2006**, *38*, 360–364. [CrossRef]
24. Harvey, D. Assessment of the flexibility of elite athletes using the modified Thomas test. *Br. J. Sports Med.* **1998**, *32*, 68–70. [CrossRef]
25. Cronin, J.; Nash, M.; Whatman, C. The acute effects of hamstring stretching and vibration on dynamic knee joint range of motion and jump performance. *Phys. Ther. Sport* **2008**, *9*, 89–96. [CrossRef]
26. Behm, D.G.; Bambury, A.; Cahill, F.; Power, K. Effect of acute static stretching on force, balance, reaction time, and movement time. *Med. Sci. Sports Exerc.* **2004**, *36*, 1397–1402. [CrossRef] [PubMed]
27. Palmieri, R.M.; Ingersoll, C.D.; Hoffman, M.A. The Hoffmann reflex: Methodologic considerations and applications for use in sports medicine and athletic training research. *J. Athl. Train.* **2004**, *39*, 268–277. [PubMed]
28. Gajewski, J.; Mazur-Różycka, J. The H-reflex as an important indicator in kinesiology. *Hum. Mov.* **2016**, *17*, 64–71. [CrossRef]
29. Park, J.; Hopkins, J.T. Induced anterior knee pain immediately reduces involuntary and voluntary quadriceps activation. *Clin. J. Sport Med.* **2013**, *23*, 19–24. [CrossRef]
30. Cohen, J. Quantitative methods in psychology: A power primer. *Psychol. Bull.* **1992**, *112*, 155–159. [CrossRef]
31. Thomas, J.; Nelson, J. *Research Methods in Physical Activity*, 5th ed.; Human Kinetics: Champaign, IL, USA, 2005; pp. 196–200.
32. Burke, D. Clinical uses of H reflexes of upper and lower limb muscles. *Clin. Neurophysiol. Pract.* **2016**, *1*, 9–17. [CrossRef] [PubMed]
33. McNeal, J.R.; Sands, W.A. Acute static stretching reduces lower extremity power in trained children. *Pediatr. Exerc. Sci.* **2003**, *15*, 139–145. [CrossRef]
34. González-Ravé, J.M.; Machado, L.; Navarro-Valdivielso, F.; Vilas-Boas, J.P. Acute effects of heavy-load exercises, stretching exercises, and heavy-load plus stretching exercises on squat jump and countermovement jump performance. *J. Strength Cond. Res.* **2009**, *23*, 472–479. [CrossRef]
35. Dalrymple, K.J.; Davis, S.E.; Dwyer, G.B.; Moir, G.L. Effect of static and dynamic stretching on vertical jump performance in collegiate women volleyball players. *J. Strength Cond. Res.* **2010**, *24*, 149–155. [CrossRef]
36. Kay, A.D.; Blazevich, A.J. Reductions in active plantar flexion moment are significantly correlated with static stretch duration. *Eur. J. Sports Sci.* **2008**, *8*, 41–46. [CrossRef]
37. McHugh, M.P.; Cosgrave, C.H. To stretch or not to stretch: The role of stretching in injury prevention and performance. *Scand. J. Med. Sci. Sports* **2010**, *20*, 169–181. [CrossRef] [PubMed]

38. Jang, H.S.; Kim, D.; Park, J. Immediate effects of different types of stretching exercises on badminton jump smash. *J. Sports Med. Phys. Fit.* **2018**, *58*, 1014–1020.
39. Brandenburg, J.; Pitney, W.A.; Luebbers, P.E.; Veera, A.; Czajka, A. Time course of changes in vertical-jumping ability after static stretching. *Int. J. Sports Physiol. Perform.* **2007**, *2*, 170–181. [CrossRef] [PubMed]
40. Samuel, M.N.; Holcomb, W.R.; Guadagnoli, M.A.; Rubley, M.D.; Wallmann, H. Acute effects of static and ballistic stretching on measures of strength and power. *J. Strength Cond. Res.* **2008**, *22*, 1422–1428. [CrossRef]
41. Pinto, M.D.; Wilhelm, E.N.; Tricoli, V.; Pinto, R.S.; Blazevich, A.J. Differential Effects of 30-vs. 60-Second Static Muscle Stretching on Vertical Jump Performance. *J. Strength Cond. Res.* **2014**, *28*, 3440–3446. [CrossRef]
42. Bogdanis, G.C.; Donti, O.; Tsolakis, C.; Smilios, I.; Bishop, D.J. Intermittent but not continuous static stretching improves subsequent vertical jump performance in flexibility-trained athletes. *J. Strength Cond. Res.* **2019**, *33*, 203–210. [CrossRef] [PubMed]
43. Kay, A.D.; Blazevich, A.J. Effect of acute static stretch on maximal muscle performance: A systematic review. *Med. Sci. Sports Exerc.* **2012**, *44*, 154–164. [CrossRef]
44. Simic, L.; Sarabon, N.; Markovic, G. Does pre-exercise static stretching inhibit maximal muscular performance? A meta-analytical review. *Scand. J. Med. Sci. Sports* **2013**, *23*, 131–148. [CrossRef]
45. Rehn, B.; Lidstrom, J.; Skoglund, J.; Lindstrom, B. Effects on leg muscular performance from whole-body vibration exercise: A systematic review. *Scand. J. Med. Sci. Sports* **2007**, *17*, 2–11. [CrossRef]
46. Latash, M.L. *Neurophysiological Basis of Movement*, 2nd ed.; Human Kinetics: Champaign, IL, USA, 2007.
47. Kröger, S.; Watkins, B. Muscle spindle function in healthy and diseased muscle. *Skelet. Muscle* **2021**, *11*, 3. [CrossRef]
48. Sharman, M.; Cresswell, A.G.; Riek, S. Proprioceptive neuromuscular facilitation stretching: Mechanisms and clincial implications. *Sports Med.* **2006**, *36*, 929–939. [CrossRef] [PubMed]
49. Burke, R.; Rudomin, P.; Zajac, F. The effect of activation history on tension production by individual muscle units. *Brain Res.* **1976**, *109*, 515–529. [CrossRef]
50. Robbins, D.W. Postactivation potentiation and its practical applicability: A brief review. *J. Strength Cond. Res.* **2005**, *19*, 453–458. [CrossRef] [PubMed]
51. Toumi, H.; Poumarat, G.; Benjamin, M.; Best, T.; F'Guyer, S.; Fairclough, J. New insights into the function of the vastus medialis with clinical implications. *Med. Sci. Sports Exerc.* **2007**, *39*, 1153–1159. [CrossRef]
52. Cowan, S.M.; Bennell, K.L.; Hodges, P.W.; Crossley, K.M.; McConnell, J. Delayed onset of electromyographic activity of vastus medialis obliquus relative to vastus lateralis in subjects with patellofemoral pain syndrome. *Arch. Phys. Med. Rehabil.* **2001**, *82*, 183–189. [CrossRef]
53. Layec, G.; Bringard, A.; Fur, Y.L.; Vilmen, C.; Micallef, J.-P.; Perrey, S.; Cozzone, P.; Bendahan, D. Effects of a prior high-intensity knee-extension exercise on muscle recruitment and energy cost: A combined local and global investigation in humans. *Exp. Physiol.* **2009**, *94*, 704–719. [CrossRef]
54. Blazevich, A.J.; Babault, N. Post-activation potentiation versus post-activation performance enhancement in humans: Historical perspective, underlying mecahnisms, and current issues. *Front. Physiol.* **2019**, *10*, 1–19. [CrossRef]
55. Trimble, M.H.; Harp, S.S. Prostexercise potentiation of the H-reflex in humans. *Med. Sci. Sports Exerc.* **1998**, *30*, 933–941.
56. Folland, J.P.; Wakamatsu, T.; Fimland, M.S. The influence of maximal isometric activity on twitch and H-reflex potentiation, and quadriceps femoris performance. *Eur. J. Appl. Physiol.* **2008**, *104*, 739–748. [CrossRef]
57. Vila-Chã, C.; Falla, D.; Correia, M.V.; Farina, D. Change in H reflex and V wave following short-term endurance and strength training. *J. Appl. Physiol.* **2012**, *112*, 54–63. [CrossRef]
58. Lima, C.D.; Brown, L.E.; Wong, M.; Levya, W.D.; Pinto, R.S.; Cadore, E.L.; Ruas, C.V. Acute effects of static vs. ballistic stretching on strength and muscular fatigue between ballet dancers and resistance trained women. *J. Strength Cond. Res.* **2016**, *30*, 3220–3227. [CrossRef] [PubMed]
59. Alrowayeh, H.N.; Sabbahi, M. Vastus medialis H-reflex reliability during standing. *J. Clin. Neurophysiol.* **2006**, *23*, 79–84. [CrossRef] [PubMed]
60. Marshall, P.W.; Rasmussen, S.B.; Krogh, M.; Halley, S.; Siegler, J.C. Changes in the quadriceps spinal-reflex pathway after repeated sprint cycling are not influenced by ischemic preconditioning. *Eur. J. Appl. Physiol.* **2020**, *120*, 1189–1202. [CrossRef] [PubMed]

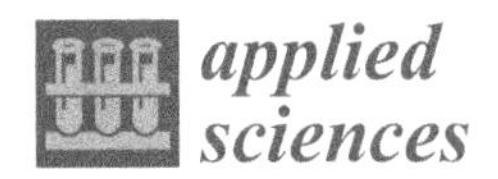

applied sciences

MDPI

Article

Effects of Obesity on Adaptation Transfer from Treadmill to Over-Ground Walking

Daekyoo Kim *, Phillip C. Desrochers, Cara L. Lewis and Simone V. Gill *

College of Health and Rehabilitation Science: Sargent College, Boston University, Boston, MA 02215, USA; pdesroch@bu.edu (P.C.D.); lewisc@bu.edu (C.L.L.)
* Correspondence: dkhy@bu.edu (D.K.); simvgill@bu.edu (S.V.G.); Tel.: +1-(617)-353-7472 (D.K.); +1-(617)-353-7513 (S.V.G.)

Abstract: Discerning whether individuals with obesity transfer walking adaptation from treadmill to over-ground walking is critical to advancing our understanding of walking adaptation and its usefulness in rehabilitating obese populations. We examined whether the aftereffects following split-belt treadmill adaptation transferred to over-ground walking in adults with normal-weight body mass index (BMI) and obese BMI. Nineteen young adults with obesity and 19 age-matched adults with normal weight walked on flat ground at their preferred speed before and after walking on a treadmill with tied belts (preferred speed) and with the split-belt at their preferred speed and at a speed 50% slower than their preferred speed. The adaptation and aftereffects in step length and double-limb support time symmetry were calculated. We found that the amount of temporal adaptation was similar for adults with obesity and with normal weight ($p > 0.05$). However, adults with obesity showed greater asymmetry for double-limb support time following split-belt treadmill walking compared to adults with normal weight ($p < 0.05$). Furthermore, the transfer of asymmetry for double-limb support time from the treadmill to over-ground walking was less in adults with obesity than in adults with normal weight ($p < 0.05$). The transfer of adapted gait following split-belt treadmill walking provides insight into how atypical walking patterns in individuals with obesity could be remediated using long-term gait training.

Keywords: obesity; gait; adaptation; rehabilitation

Citation: Kim, D.; Desrochers, P.C.; Lewis, C.L.; Gill, S.V. Effects of Obesity on Adaptation Transfer from Treadmill to Over-Ground Walking. *Appl. Sci.* **2021**, *11*, 2108. https://doi.org/10.3390/app11052108

Academic Editor: Nyeonju Kang

Received: 22 January 2021
Accepted: 22 February 2021
Published: 27 February 2021

1. Introduction

Obesity is a public health epidemic, elevating the risk of numerous comorbid conditions, including heart disease, stroke, type 2 diabetes, and certain cancers that may cause premature death [1]. The prevalence of obesity in the United States is 42.4% among adults over 20 years old and has increased 12% over the past 20 years [2]. To combat obesity, increasing energy expenditure via increasing physical activity has been strongly recommended; physical activity promotes weight loss and can help maintain cardiovascular and metabolic health [3]. Unfortunately, individuals with obesity fall short of physical activity recommendations [4]. Although walking is a recommended and cost-effective intervention used to increase overall physical activity, walking may be harmful to individuals with obesity [5]. Common characteristics of individuals with obesity include altered spatiotemporal gait parameters (slower speed and shorter and wider steps) and joint kinematics (less flexed lower extremity joints) compared to adults with normal weight [6–8], which likely serve as ways to compensate for a lack of postural stability [9].

Obesity is associated with the abnormal distribution of body fat in the abdominal area and greater thigh and trunk girth [5,10,11], which could hinder the ability to adapt walking patterns to changes caused by environmental constraints, such as surfaces with obstacles or slopes [12]. A failure to quickly and effectively adapt to change while walking can lead to injuries and poses a safety risk [13]. For example, compared to normal-weight adults, adults with obesity demonstrate poor strategies during obstacle avoidance, with higher toe clearance to cross low versus high obstacles [14]. Additionally, adults with obesity have difficulty matching steps to an audio metronome beat while walking; they step later than the metronome beat regardless of the BPM (beats per minute) [12]. Adults with obesity also walk slower after a slow metronome pace and faster after a fast metronome pace, thus demonstrating aftereffects. Taken together, the evidence shows that these challenges with adaptation may make it difficult to safely complete walking and activities of daily living, such as walking to the grocery store and crossing the street in accordance with traffic signals. This raises a question; how do individuals with obesity change the ways in which they walk when posed with a disruption in their typical patterns of walking?

A split-belt treadmill training paradigm has been used to examine walking adaptation. In a split-belt treadmill paradigm, two separate belts moving beneath each leg can be independently controlled [15,16]. This paradigm allows for repeated practice of walking in which each leg moves at a different speed. Previous research on split-belt treadmill walking adaptation in healthy adults has demonstrated that step length and double-limb support time are asymmetric during an initial adaptation period when the belt speed is changed so that one belt moves faster than the other [16]. Consequently, the limb on the slow belt takes a longer step than the limb walking on the fast belt. Over time, walkers gradually adapt to re-establish step symmetry during split-belt walking. After only 10–15 min of split-belt treadmill walking, walkers exhibit aftereffects [16,17]. These findings have led to the suggestion that the adaptive strategies observed during split-belt treadmill walking may have the potential to be used as a rehabilitative technique for individuals post-stroke [16,18], with Parkinson's disease [19], and who have had amputations [20]. However, whether the same would be true for adults with obesity is unknown. Using split-belt treadmill training as a rehabilitative tool might spur faster adaptation to future perturbations experienced in everyday life and facilitate increased physical activity; short-term changes in walking could be capitalized upon with repeated practice to produce long-term changes in walking [21].

Critical to advancing our understanding of gait adaptation and its usefulness in rehabilitating obese populations is discerning whether the adaptive effects observed on a treadmill transfer to over-ground walking. Previous studies demonstrated the transfer of split-belt treadmill walking adaptation to over-ground walking [21]. The results revealed that the adapted walking pattern following split-belt treadmill walking partially transfers to over-ground in healthy young adults, suggesting that the treadmill walking adaptation influenced some aspects of over-ground walking. Examining whether adults with obesity transfer walking from the treadmill to over-ground walking could provide support for the usefulness of treadmill walking as a rehabilitative tool.

Therefore, the current study investigated the effects of obesity on adaptation and transfer from the treadmill to over-ground walking. We hypothesized that normal and obese BMI groups would successfully adapt both spatial and temporal parameters following split-belt perturbations and would transfer adapted walking patterns from the split-belt treadmill to over-ground walking. We also hypothesized that the extent of the adaptation and transfer would be less in adults with obesity than in adults with normal weight [12–14].

2. Materials and Methods

2.1. Participants

Thirty-eight young adults (19 normal weight BMI and 19 obese BMI) participated in this study (Table 1). The study eligibility criteria included being between 18–35 years old, having no weight loss surgery, having no significant cardiovascular, vestibular, or other neurologic disorders, having no hip, knee, or foot pain on most days during the past 90 days, and having the ability to walk independently on a treadmill for over 40 min. All the participants gave informed written consent before participating. The Boston University Institutional Review Board approved the protocols (4922E).

Table 1. Demographics and anthropometric information. Means are listed with standard deviations in parentheses.

	BMI Groups	
	[1] NW (N = 19; [3] F = 10)	[2] OB (N = 19; [3] F = 12)
Age (years)	23.21 (5.46)	28.27 (4.03)
Height (m)	1.71 (0.09)	1.69 (0.08)
Weight (kg)	66.83 (12.46)	119.74 (29.08)
BMI (kg/m^2)	22.37 (2.49)	42.62 (8.01)
Waist Circumference (cm)	78.93 (9.01)	123.56 (18.42)
Gait Velocity (m/s)	1.24 (0.12)	1.05 (0.12)

[1] NW: normal weight; [2] OB: obesity; [3] F: female.

2.2. Experimental Protocol

Spatiotemporal walking data were collected at the Motor Development Lab and the Human Adaptation Lab in Sargent College, Boston University, Boston, MA, from July 2019 through to November 2019. Walking adaptation was characterized using a 6.10 m long × 0.89 m wide pressure-sensitive gait carpet (Protokinetics, LLC; Peekskill, NY, USA; 120 Hz sampling frequency) and a split-belt treadmill with two independent belts and full-length force plates (Bertec Corporation, Columbus, OH; 1000 Hz sampling frequency). As these data were collected as part of a larger study evaluating navicular drop, the participants walked barefoot with stick-on foot pads throughout the experiment. The experimental paradigm is shown in Figure 1. The walking task involved six conditions. In the first condition, participants walked on the carpet at their own pace for two minutes. Participants began the trials standing 2 m before the edge of the carpet and ended the trials 2 m after walking off the carpet. Trials began and ended the walking with verbal prompts from the experimenter (i.e., "Go" and "Stop"). After that, they turned around and walked again. The participants' comfortable over-ground walking speeds were calculated by the total step length divided by the total step time (m/s) in the first over-ground condition. This was used to set the preferred walking speed in the following treadmill conditions. The participants then moved to the treadmill and performed four treadmill walking conditions (Figure 1). As the treadmill speed was constant within each of the four treadmill walking conditions, the transition phases between tied-belt and split-belt were discarded for the analysis. All the participants reported that their dominant leg was the right leg. During treadmill walking conditions, participants were positioned in the middle of the treadmill with their dominant leg on the right-side belt (the slow belt was always on the dominant leg). Participants were instructed to refrain from looking down at the belts. The treadmill had rails on the front, left, and right sides to grab in case they lost balance, but participants were instructed not to grab the rails unless they felt unbalanced. Before testing, all participants walked on a treadmill at their comfortable walking speed until they felt comfortable with treadmill walking and ready for testing. Participants initially performed a tied-belt walking condition for five minutes. During the tied-belt condition, the treadmill belt speeds were set at each participant's preferred over-ground walking speed. Following this, the participants underwent a split-belt condition for 10 min. During the split-belt condition, the belt under the left leg moved at the participant's preferred speed while the belt under the right leg moved at a speed 50% slower than their preferred speed. As has been demonstrated previously [15,17,22], this split-belt perturbation typically causes spatial and temporal gait asymmetries (i.e., visible interlimb difference); however, with 10 min of practice with 'split-belts', gait symmetry is typically restored and the asymmetric stepping goes away. Following this split-belt condition, the participants walked on tied-belts for 5 min to wash out the perturbation. At the beginning of the washout condition, the participants typically exhibit the opposite asymmetry in their gait (i.e., they walk with an inter-limb difference in the opposite direction). Thus, we assessed the storage and retention of the novel walking pattern in the washout condition. By the end of the washout condition, the participants returned to symmetrical walking on the tied-belts. Participants then performed a second split-belt perturbation condition for five minutes to examine how quickly they re-adapted during split-belt walking. Following this, the participants completed an over-ground walking condition again at their own pace for two minutes (Figure 1).

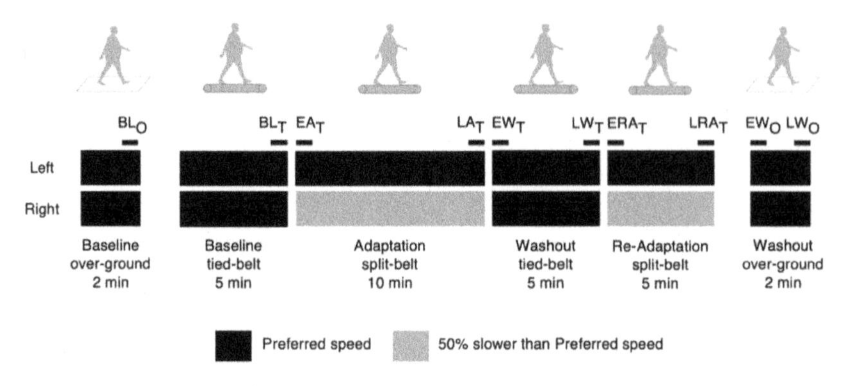

Figure 1. Time course for the experimental paradigm showing the over-ground baseline (BL_O), treadmill baseline (BL_T), split-belt treadmill adaptation (EA_T & LA_T), tied-belt treadmill washout (EW_T & LW_T), split-belt treadmill re-adaptation (ERA_T & LRA_T), and over-ground washout conditions (EW_O & LW_O). For split-belt treadmill walking, the upper bar shows fast (left, black) belt speed and the lower bar shows slow (right, gray) belt speed.

2.3. Data Analysis

We examined where the participants placed their feet (spatial coordination) and when participants placed their feet as they walked (temporal coordination) during all of the testing conditions. Center of pressure (COP) data were determined using the pressure-sensitive gait carpet for over-ground walking and the force plates for treadmill walking. COP consisted of a time series of the x and y coordinates. Gait events, such as heel strike and toe-off, were independently determined for each leg from the pressure data for over-ground walking and the force data for treadmill walking. The step length (m) was calculated by the absolute difference in the anteroposterior center of pressure (COP) position between the right and left foot at the heel strike. Double-limb support time (s) was measured by the period between the heel strike and the contralateral toe-off for each step. Step length symmetry was calculated as the ratio of the slow (right; dominant leg) step length to the fast (left; non-dominant leg) step length. Double-limb support symmetry was calculated as the ratio of the initial double-limb support time of the slow (right) leg to that of the fast (left) leg over the gait cycle. Positive symmetry values indicate a longer left step length and initial double-limb support time, while negative values indicate a shorter right step length and initial double-limb support time. A value of 0 indicates perfect symmetry, and with a greater symmetry value, the gait is more asymmetric. To determine the transfer of aftereffects observed on the treadmill to over-ground walking, we calculated a transfer index [21]:

$$\text{Transfer Index} = \frac{EW_O - BL_O}{EW_T - BL_T},$$

where EW_O is the mean of the first ten strides in the over-ground washout condition, BL_O is the mean of the first 10 strides in the over-ground baseline condition, EW_T is the mean of the first 10 strides in the tied-belt treadmill washout, and BL_T is the mean of the first 10 strides in the tied-belt treadmill baseline condition.

2.4. Statistical Analysis

Two-way repeated measures analysis of variance (ANOVA) was used to identify statistically significant interactions in the gait symmetry (i.e., step length symmetry and double-limb support time symmetry) between groups (i.e., adults with obesity vs. adults with normal weight) across testing conditions. To test the degree of adaptation during the split-belt treadmill walking, we compared gait symmetry between groups and between adaptation conditions (tied-belt treadmill baseline (BL_T) vs. early split-belt treadmill adaptation (EA_T)). To test storage (what participants learned) during the adaptation period, we compared gait symmetry between groups and between the washout condition (tied-belt treadmill baseline (BL_T) vs. the early tied-belt treadmill washout (EW_T)). To test the memory of the adapted walking pattern when re-exposed to the same perturbation, we compared gait symmetry between groups and between the re-adaptation condition (early split-belt treadmill adaptation (EA_T) vs. the early split-belt treadmill re-adaptation (ERA_T)). When the ANOVA yielded significant results, post hoc analyses were performed using a Bonferroni correction. Lastly, to test the transfer of aftereffect (i.e., how split-belt training influenced participants' abilities to store a new walking pattern) from the treadmill to over-ground walking, we used a t-test to compare the transfer index between the groups. The values for each outcome variable were averaged over the first 10 strides in EA_T, EW_T, ERA_T, and EW_O, as well as the last 10 steps in BL_O, BL_T, LA_T, LW_T, LRA_T, and LW_O. The effect sizes for the ANOVA were reported via partial eta squared (ηp^2) after p-values, giving 0.01 (small), 0.09 (medium), and 0.25 (large) effects. Effect sizes for the t-test were reported via Cohen's d considering 0.2 (small), 0.5 (medium), and 0.8 (large) effects [23]. For all tests, the statistical significance was set at 0.05 (two-tailed). All the statistical analyses were performed using SPSS (Version 26.0, SPSS Inc., Chicago, IL, USA).

3. Results

Figure 2 shows changes in double-limb support time symmetry (Figure 2a) and step length symmetry (Figure 2c) over the course of over-ground and split-belt treadmill walking. There was no statistically significant interaction between the groups and the adaptation conditions on double-limb support time symmetry ($F(1, 72) = 0.01$, $p = 0.94$, $\eta p^2 < 0.01$; Figure 2b) and step length symmetry ($F(1, 72) = 0.17$, $p = 0.68$, $\eta p^2 < 0.01$; Figure 2d). The main effect of the groups showed no significant difference in double-limb support time symmetry ($F(1, 72) = 0.66$, $p = 0.42$, $\eta p^2 < 0.01$) and step length symmetry ($F(1, 72) = 0.30$, $p = 0.59$, $\eta p^2 < 0.01$). The main effect of the adaptation condition showed that there were significant differences in double-limb support time symmetry ($F(1, 72) = 197.59$, $p < 0.01$, $\eta p^2 = 0.70$) and step length symmetry ($F(1, 72) = 961.74$, $p < 0.01$, $\eta p^2 = 0.92$) between the tied-belt treadmill baseline (BL_T) and early split-belt treadmill adaptation (EA_T), indicating that both groups were perturbed when the belts were first split (i.e., walking asymmetrically with inter-limb difference).

There was a statistically significant interaction between the groups and washout conditions on double-limb support time symmetry ($F(1, 72) = 5.68$, $p = 0.02$, $\eta p^2 = 0.10$; Figure 2b). The symmetry value for the double-limb support time was significantly greater in adults with obesity than in adults with normal weight during the early tied-belt washout period (when the split-belt perturbation is removed). The symmetry value for the double-limb support time was similar between adults with obesity and adults with normal weight during tied-belt baseline. There was no significant interaction between the groups and washout conditions regarding step length symmetry ($F(1, 72) = 2.91$, $p = 0.09$, $\eta p^2 = 0.03$; Figure 2d). The main effect of the group showed no significant difference in step length symmetry between adults with obesity and adults with normal weight ($F(1, 72) = 2.39$, $p = 0.13$, $\eta p^2 = 0.02$). The main effect of the washout condition showed that there was a significant difference in step length symmetry between the tied-belt treadmill baseline (BL_T) and the early tied-belt treadmill washout (EW_T) ($F(1, 72) = 241.95$, $p < 0.01$, $\eta p^2 = 0.74$), indicating that both groups showed aftereffects (i.e., walking asymmetrically with inter-limb difference in the opposite direction).

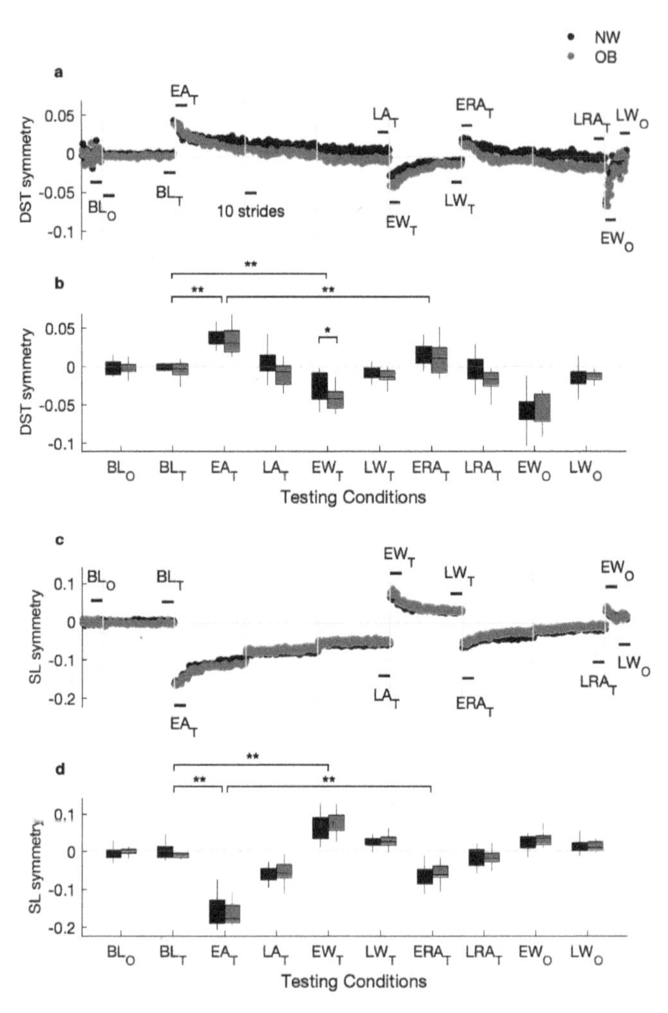

Figure 2. Experimental paradigm showing the periods of testing conditions in a light gray vertical line: over-ground baseline (BL_O), treadmill baseline (BL_T), early treadmill adaptation (EA_T), late treadmill adaptation (LA_T), early treadmill washout (EW_T), late treadmill washout (LW_T), early treadmill re-adaptation (ERA_T), late treadmill re-adaptation (LRA_T), early over-ground washout (EW_O), late over-ground washout (LW_O). Double-limb support time (DST) symmetry (**a**) and step length (SL) symmetry (**c**) values for sequential strides over the ground and on the treadmill between adults with normal weight (dark grey) and obesity (dark brown) across all testing conditions. A value of 0, represented as a light gray horizontal axis, indicates perfect symmetry. Means and standard errors for DST symmetry (**b**) and SL symmetry (**d**) are shown between the body mass index (BMI) groups (NW: normal weight; OB: obesity) across testing conditions. ** $p < 0.01$; * $p < 0.05$.

There was no statistically significant interaction between the groups and re-adaptation conditions on double-limb support time symmetry ($F(1, 72) = 0.62$, $p = 0.43$, $\eta p^2 < 0.01$; Figure 2b) and step length symmetry ($F(1, 72) = 1.01$, $p = 0.32$, $\eta p^2 = 0.01$; Figure 2d). The main effect of the group showed no significant difference in double-limb support time symmetry ($F(1, 72) = 0.18$, $p = 0.19$, $\eta p^2 = 0.02$) and step length symmetry ($F(1, 72) = 0.06$, $p = 0.81$, $\eta p^2 < 0.01$). The main effect of the adaptation condition showed that there were significant differences in double-limb support time symmetry ($F(1, 72) = 37.10$, $p < 0.01$, $\eta p^2 = 0.31$)

and step length symmetry ($F(1, 72) = 250.91$, $p < 0.01$, $\eta p^2 = 0.75$) between the early split-belt treadmill adaptation (EA_T) and the early split-belt treadmill re-adaptation (ERA_T), indicating that both groups experienced smaller errors early in the re-adaptation period rather than early in the initial adaptation period (i.e., participants were less perturbed by the split-belts).

Figure 3 shows that there was a significant difference in the transfer of double-limb support time symmetry (from the treadmill to over-ground walking) between groups. The transfer index for double-limb support time symmetry was less in adults with obesity than in adults with normal weight ($t(36) = 3.49$, $p < 0.01$, $d = 0.75$; Figure 3b). However, the transfer index for step length symmetry was not statistically different in adults with obesity compared to adults with normal weight ($t(36) = 0.58$, $p = 0.15$, $d = 0.17$; Figure 3a).

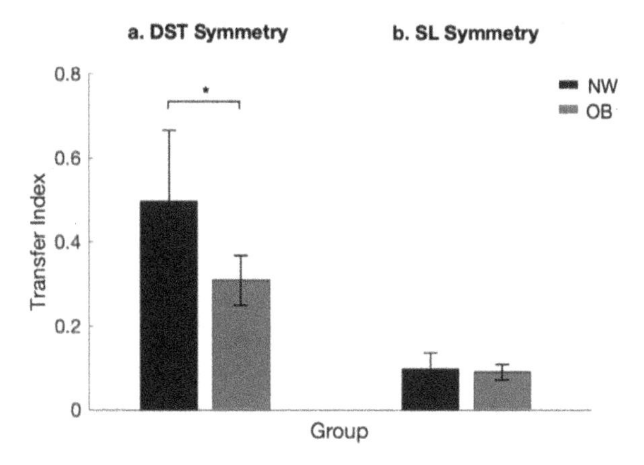

Figure 3. Transfer Index for adults with normal weight (dark grey) and obesity (dark brown) for double-limb support time (DST) symmetry (**a**) and step length (SL) symmetry (**b**). The transfer index indicates the amount of adaptation transfer from the treadmill to over-ground walking in each BMI group. For both adapted parameters, the transfer index is greater in adults with normal weight than in adults with obesity. Error bars indicate the standard deviation. Asterisk indicates a significant difference between groups. * $p < 0.05$.

4. Discussion

In the current study, we demonstrated that the temporal gait adaptation following split-belt treadmill walking was greater in adults with obesity versus adults with normal weight. We also found that a temporal gait adaptation following split-belt treadmill walking transfers to over-ground walking in both adults with obesity and adults with normal weight. The adaptation transfer of double-limb support time was smaller in adults with obesity when compared with the adults with normal weight. This provides additional support for the previous suggestion that gait characteristics such as lower step frequency and longer double-limb support phase exist in those with obesity.

Throughout the adaptation, we observed that both groups successfully adapted their walking patterns to split-belt perturbations (adaptation), showed aftereffects (washout), and saved the memory of adapted walking patterns (re-adaptation), which is supported by previous research focusing on healthy young adults [16,17,22]. This is the first study, however, to demonstrate that adults with obesity adapted their walking and transferred from the treadmill to a real-world task: in this case, over-ground walking. In the current study, step length and double support asymmetries following split-belt treadmill adaptation transferred to over-ground walking. Therefore, this study supports the possibility of using a treadmill to, for instance, lengthen or quicken stepping movements or manage new constraints in individuals with obesity.

Contrary to our hypothesis, however, we did not observe any differences in step length symmetry between normal-weight adults and adults with obesity throughout the testing conditions. One interpretation is that the amounts of adaptation, aftereffects, savings, and transfers for step length symmetry may depend on the imposed walking speed as a mediator of the effect of obesity on gait symmetry. In the current study, to maximize the effect of obesity on gait adaptation, treadmill belt speeds were set at each participant's preferred over-ground walking speed. Specifically, each participant's treadmill baseline walking speed was matched with their self-selected comfortable walking speed over the ground, which is more like everyday life where speed is sometimes imposed. However, we acknowledge that using a preferred speed for each participant may have limited the amount of variability in response to the split-belt perturbation. Given that each participant walked at a comfortable speed and adapted to the split-belt perturbation with a 2:1 speed ratio between the fast and slow belt, this explains how participants with obesity adapted and washed out at similar rates to participants with normal weight despite a slower walking speed. Future research may elucidate whether a fixed split-belt speed ratio may affect the rate of adaptation (split-belt) and de-adaptation (tied-belt) across BMI groups.

Interestingly, the initial double-limb support times of both the slow (right) leg and the fast (left) leg over the gait cycle were larger in adults with obesity versus adults with normal weight over all of the testing conditions. This finding suggests that temporal gait is affected by obesity, which is consistent with previous findings [5,6,12]. Researchers suggest that prioritizing postural stability is likely primary for adults who have less ability to recover from a loss of balance [24]. Considering that individuals with obesity have impaired postural control and stability [25], increasing double-limb support time, along with increasing step width and decreasing walking speed, could be a primary strategy to maximize postural stability, and to avoid asymmetric gait and falling after split-belt treadmill walking. Furthermore, it is reasonable to suppose that step length could be balanced by contributions from increased double-limb support time. When exposed to split-belt perturbation, the treadmill powers the legs, so more control is required for regulating the period of double-limb support (i.e., when both limbs are on the ground). This may have led to longer double-limb support times in adults with obesity compared with adults with normal weight.

Researchers have studied how human actions adapted to a specific environment are transferred to other environments and demonstrated that similarity of the movements can influence the transfer of action [26,27]. The transfer of adapted patterns is greatest when walking in a familiar environment [28–30]. The amount of transfer could be similar for adults with obesity and with normal weight if both groups have experience with treadmill walking. We suspect that the transfer of the adapted gait pattern observed in adults with obesity could be similar to that observed in normal weight adults, considering the fact that treadmills have been widely used for exercise. However, the altered temporal gait parameters (i.e., increased double-limb support times) observed in the obese population might reduce the ability to switch temporal patterns with the change in gait environment from the treadmill to over-ground walking (i.e., less transfer of aftereffects for the temporal gait parameter).

Previous studies on rehabilitative gait training have demonstrated that, although a little different, there are similarities observed between treadmill and over-ground walking in young adults [31–33]. An ideal rehabilitation intervention could include both treadmill and over-ground walking to maximize improvements in walking through task-specific training. In the current study, participants reduced step asymmetry in both treadmill and over-ground walking and transferred aftereffects for step symmetry from the treadmill to over-ground walking. Therefore, it could be beneficial for future studies to examine the use of split-belt treadmill walking paired with over-ground walking in interventions with those with obesity. One drawback of this approach, of course, would be the cost incurred by using a rehabilitation paradigm that necessitates the use of split-belt treadmill technology. However, future findings may reveal whether there are rehabilitative benefits that outweigh the cost of the equipment.

We acknowledge that the present study has limitations. Firstly, we intentionally recruited participants without comorbidities, such as osteoarthritis, plantar fasciitis, or cardiovascular disease. Thus, the generalizability of our study is limited by the fact that our participants may not be representative of those with obesity and additional conditions. However, this reduced confounding variables that could have influenced the interpretation of our results. Secondly, the number of male participants with obesity that we tested was smaller than the number of females, which may reduce the ability to generalize the results to males. Third, we did not have the participants rate their perceived exertion during the walking task. Future studies should examine how perceived exertion affects walking adaptation in adults with obesity. Despite these limitations, our results provide important information about the effect of obesity on walking adaptation and transfer from treadmill to over-ground walking.

5. Conclusions

Our findings suggest that adults with obesity showed greater asymmetry for double-limb support time than adults with normal weight. The transfer of asymmetry for double-limb support time from the treadmill to over-ground walking was less in adults with obesity than in adults with normal weight. Understanding how individuals with obesity adapt their walking to a new environment and how adapted patterns transfer from treadmill to over-ground walking can be used to design interventions aimed at increasing physical activity.

Author Contributions: Conceptualization, D.K., C.L.L., and S.V.G.; methodology, D.K.; formal analysis, D.K.; writing—original draft preparation, D.K.; writing—review and editing, C.L.L., P.C.D., and S.V.G.; visualization, D.K.; supervision, S.V.G.; project administration, S.V.G. All authors have read and agreed to the published version of the manuscript.

Funding: This research received no external funding.

Institutional Review Board Statement: The study was conducted according to the guidelines of the Declaration of Helsinki, and approved by the Institutional Review Board of Boston University (4922E; October 15, 2019).

Informed Consent Statement: Informed consent was obtained from all subjects involved in the study. Written informed consent has been obtained from the patient(s) to publish this paper.

Data Availability Statement: The data presented in this study are available on request from the corresponding author. The data are not publicly available due to the consent provided by participants on the use of confidential data.

Conflicts of Interest: The authors declare no conflict of interest.

References

1. Jensen, M.D.; Ryan, D.H.; Apovian, C.M.; Ard, J.D.; Comuzzie, A.G.; Donato, K.A.; Hu, F.B.; Hubbard, V.S.; Jakicic, J.M.; Kushner, R.F. 2013 AHA/ACC/TOS Guideline for the Management of Overweight and Obesity in Adults: A Report of the American College of Cardiology/American Heart Association Task Force on Practice Guidelines and The Obesity Society. *J. Am. Coll. Cardiol.* **2014**, *63*, 2985–3023. [CrossRef] [PubMed]
2. Hales, C.M.; Carroll, M.D.; Fryar, C.D.; Ogden, C.L. *Prevalence of Obesity and Severe Obesity among Adults: United States, 2017–2018*; 2020. Available online: https://www.cdc.gov/nchs/products/databriefs/db360.htm (accessed on 26 February 2021).
3. World Health Organization. *Global Recommendations on Physical Activity for Health*; World Health Organization: Geneva, Switzerland, 2010.
4. Blanchard, C.M.; McGannon, K.R.; Spence, J.C.; Rhodes, R.E.; Nehl, E.; Baker, F.; Bostwick, J. Social Ecological Correlates of Physical Activity in Normal Weight, Overweight, and Obese Individuals. *Int. J. Obes.* **2005**, *29*, 720–726. [CrossRef] [PubMed]
5. Browning, R.C. Locomotion Mechanics in Obese Adults and Children. *Curr. Obes. Rep.* **2012**, *1*, 152–159. [CrossRef]
6. Kim, D.; Gill, S.V. Changes in Center of Pressure Velocities during Obstacle Crossing One Year after Bariatric Surgery. *Gait Posture* **2020**, *76*, 377–381. [CrossRef]
7. DeVita, P.; Hortobágyi, T. Obesity Is Not Associated with Increased Knee Joint Torque and Power during Level Walking. *J. Biomech.* **2003**, *36*, 1355–1362. [CrossRef]

8. Agostini, V.; Gastaldi, L.; Rosso, V.; Knaflitz, M.; Tadano, S. A Wearable Magneto-Inertial System for Gait Analysis (H-Gait): Validation on Normal Weight and Overweight/Obese Young Healthy Adults. *Sensors* **2017**, *17*, 2406. [CrossRef] [PubMed]
9. Hills, A.P.; Hennig, E.M.; Byrne, N.M.; Steele, J.R. The Biomechanics of Adiposity–Structural and Functional Limitations of Obesity and Implications for Movement. *Obes. Rev.* **2002**, *3*, 35–43. [CrossRef]
10. Alonso, A.C.; Luna, N.M.S.; Mochizuki, L.; Barbieri, F.; Santos, S.; Greve, J.M.D. The Influence of Anthropometric Factors on Postural Balance: The Relationship between Body Composition and Posturographic Measurements in Young Adults. *Clinics* **2012**, *67*, 1433–1441. [CrossRef]
11. Gill, S.V.; Hicks, G.E.; Zhang, Y.; Niu, J.; Apovian, C.M.; White, D.K. The Association of Waist Circumference with Walking Difficulty among Adults with or at Risk of Knee Osteoarthritis: The Osteoarthritis Initiative. *Osteoarthr. Cartil.* **2017**, *25*, 60–66. [CrossRef]
12. Gill, S.V. The Impact of Weight Classification on Safety: Timing Steps to Adapt to External Constraints. *J. Musculoskelet. Neuronal Interact.* **2015**, *15*, 103.
13. Hung, Y.-C.; Gill, S.V.; Meredith, G.S. Influence of Dual-Task Constraints on Whole-Body Organization during Walking in Children Who Are Overweight and Obese. *Am. J. Phys. Med. Rehabil.* **2013**, *92*, 461–471. [CrossRef]
14. Gill, S.V.; Hung, Y.-C. Effects of Overweight and Obese Body Mass on Motor Planning and Motor Skills during Obstacle Crossing in Children. *Res. Dev. Disabil.* **2014**, *35*, 46–53. [CrossRef]
15. Choi, J.T.; Bastian, A.J. Adaptation Reveals Independent Control Networks for Human Walking. *Nat. Neurosci.* **2007**, *10*, 1055–1062. [CrossRef]
16. Reisman, D.S.; Block, H.J.; Bastian, A.J. Interlimb Coordination during Locomotion: What Can Be Adapted and Stored? *J. Neurophysiol.* **2005**, *94*, 2403–2415. [CrossRef] [PubMed]
17. Malone, L.A.; Bastian, A.J. Thinking about Walking: Effects of Conscious Correction versus Distraction on Locomotor Adaptation. *J. Neurophysiol.* **2010**, *103*, 1954–1962. [CrossRef]
18. Reisman, D.S.; Wityk, R.; Silver, K.; Bastian, A.J. Locomotor Adaptation on a Split-Belt Treadmill Can Improve Walking Symmetry Post-Stroke. *Brain* **2007**, *130*, 1861–1872. [CrossRef]
19. Roemmich, R.T.; Nocera, J.R.; Stegemöller, E.L.; Hassan, A.; Okun, M.S.; Hass, C.J. Locomotor Adaptation and Locomotor Adaptive Learning in Parkinson's Disease and Normal Aging. *Clin. Neurophysiol.* **2014**, *125*, 313–319. [CrossRef]
20. Selgrade, B.P.; Toney, M.E.; Chang, Y.-H. Two Biomechanical Strategies for Locomotor Adaptation to Split-Belt Treadmill Walking in Subjects with and without Transtibial Amputation. *J. Biomech.* **2017**, *53*, 136–143. [CrossRef] [PubMed]
21. Reisman, D.S.; Wityk, R.; Silver, K.; Bastian, A.J. Split-Belt Treadmill Adaptation Transfers to Overground Walking in Persons Poststroke. *Neurorehabilit. Neural Repair* **2009**, *23*, 735–744. [CrossRef] [PubMed]
22. Mawase, F.; Haizler, T.; Bar-Haim, S.; Karniel, A. Kinetic Adaptation during Locomotion on a Split-Belt Treadmill. *J. Neurophysiol.* **2013**, *109*, 2216–2227. [CrossRef] [PubMed]
23. Sawilowsky, S.S. New Effect Size Rules of Thumb. *J. Mod. Appl. Stat. Methods* **2009**, *8*, 26. [CrossRef]
24. Bruijn, S.M.; Van Dieën, J.H. Control of Human Gait Stability through Foot Placement. *J. R. Soc. Interface* **2018**, *15*, 20170816. [CrossRef] [PubMed]
25. Forhan, M.; Gill, S.V. Obesity, Functional Mobility and Quality of Life. *Best Pract. Res. Clin. Endocrinol. Metab.* **2013**, *27*, 129–137. [CrossRef] [PubMed]
26. Krakauer, J.W.; Mazzoni, P.; Ghazizadeh, A.; Ravindran, R.; Shadmehr, R. Generalization of Motor Learning Depends on the History of Prior Action. *PLoS Biol.* **2006**, *4*, e316. [CrossRef]
27. Morton, S.M.; Bastian, A.J. Prism Adaptation during Walking Generalizes to Reaching and Requires the Cerebellum. *J. Neurophysiol.* **2004**, *92*, 2497–2509. [CrossRef]
28. Anstis, S. Aftereffects from Jogging. *Exp. Brain Res.* **1995**, *103*, 476–478. [CrossRef]
29. Earhart, G.M.; Melvill Jones, G.; Horak, F.B.; Block, E.W.; Weber, K.D.; Fletcher, W.A. Transfer of Podokinetic Adaptation from Stepping to Hopping. *J. Neurophysiol.* **2002**, *87*, 1142–1144. [CrossRef] [PubMed]
30. Reynolds, R.F.; Bronstein, A.M. The Moving Platform Aftereffect: Limited Generalization of a Locomotor Adaptation. *J. Neurophysiol.* **2004**, *91*, 92–100. [CrossRef] [PubMed]
31. Hollman, J.H.; Watkins, M.K.; Imhoff, A.C.; Braun, C.E.; Akervik, K.A.; Ness, D.K. A Comparison of Variability in Spatiotemporal Gait Parameters between Treadmill and Overground Walking Conditions. *Gait Posture* **2016**, *43*, 204–209. [CrossRef]
32. Parvataneni, K.; Ploeg, L.; Olney, S.J.; Brouwer, B. Kinematic, Kinetic and Metabolic Parameters of Treadmill versus Overground Walking in Healthy Older Adults. *Clin. Biomech.* **2009**, *24*, 95–100. [CrossRef]
33. Riley, P.O.; Paolini, G.; Della Croce, U.; Paylo, K.W.; Kerrigan, D.C. A Kinematic and Kinetic Comparison of Overground and Treadmill Walking in Healthy Subjects. *Gait Posture* **2007**, *26*, 17–24. [CrossRef] [PubMed]

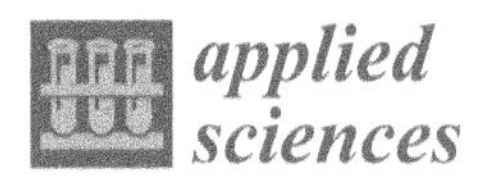

MDPI

Article

Foot Contact Dynamics and Fall Risk among Children Diagnosed with Idiopathic Toe Walking

Rahul Soangra [1,2], Michael Shiraishi [1], Richard Beuttler [3], Michelle Gwerder [3], LouAnne Boyd [4], Venkatesan Muthukumar [5], Mohamed Trabia [5], Afshin Aminian [6] and Marybeth Grant-Beuttler [1,6,*]

1 Crean College of Health and Behavioral Sciences, Chapman University, Orange, CA 92866, USA; soangra@chapman.edu (R.S.); shiraishi@chapman.edu (M.S.)
2 Fowler School of Engineering, Chapman University, Orange, CA 92866, USA
3 School of Pharmacy, Chapman University, Orange, CA 92618, USA; rbeuttle@chapman.edu (R.B.); michelle.gwerder@hest.ethz.ch (M.G.)
4 Institute of Biomechanics, 8092 ETH Zurich, Switzerland; lboyd@chapman.edu
5 Howard R. Hughes College of Engineering, University of Nevada, Las Vegas, NV 89154, USA; Venkatesan.muthukumar@unlv.edu (V.M.); Mohamed.trabia@unlv.edu (M.T.)
6 Children's Hospital of Orange County, Orange, CA 92868, USA; aaminian@choc.org
* Correspondence: beuttler@chapman.edu; Tel.: +1-714-744-7626

Abstract: Children that are diagnosed with Idiopathic Toe walking (cITW) are characterized by persistent toe-to-toe contacts. The objective of this study was to explore whether typical foot contact dynamics during walking predisposes cITW to a higher risk of falling. Twenty cITW and age-matched controls performed typical and toe walking trials. The gait parameters related to foot contact dynamics, vertical force impulses during stance, slip, and trip risk were compared for both groups. We found that cITW manifest less stable gait and produced significantly higher force impulses during push-off. Additionally, we found that cITW had a higher slip-initiation risk that was associated with higher foot contact horizontal and vertical velocities in addition to lower transitional acceleration of center of mass. We found that cITW exhibited a higher trip risk with toe clearance being significantly lower when compared to healthy counterparts. This study allowed for a quantitative description of foot contact dynamics and delineated typical from toe walking among cITW. Overall, the results indicate that cITW are less stable during typical walking and are prone to a higher risk of slip and trip-like falls.

Keywords: Idiopathic Toe Walking; fall risk; foot contact dynamics; foot initial contact; push-off

Citation: Soangra, R.; Shiraishi, M.; Beuttler, R.; Gwerder, M.; Boyd, L.; Muthukumar, V.; Trabia, M.; Aminian, A.; Grant-Beuttler, M. Foot Contact Dynamics and Fall Risk among Children Diagnosed with Idiopathic Toe Walking. *Appl. Sci.* **2021**, *11*, 2862. https://doi.org/10.3390/app11062862

Academic Editor: Nyeonju Kang

Received: 1 February 2021
Accepted: 18 March 2021
Published: 23 March 2021

1. Introduction

Toe walking is defined as walking on the forefeet as compared to a typical heel-toe gait pattern. Toe touch can be observed in early ambulation, but it is considered to be atypical after three years [1,2]. The prevalence of Idiopathic Toe Walking (ITW) among children has been reported between 2–12 % of the child population [3]. Earlier research has reported an increased fall risk due to frequent tripping and pain in the leg or foot among children diagnosed with Idiopathic Toe Walking (cITW) [1,4]. Some researchers also reported limited ankle dorsiflexion, functional and passive range-of-motion (ROM), which predisposes them to higher fall risk and ankle injuries [5]. The cause of toe walking in ITW may not be clear. However, some researchers emphasize hyperactive reflexes and they have based current therapeutic strategies on this theory in the clinics [6–8].

Clinicians and movement science researchers have sought to understand how toe walking behavior influences fall risk by monitoring the subtle differences in the ground reaction forces (GRF). GRF metrics may reflect internal loading differences among cITW as compared to healthy controls. Toe walking with GRF analysis can potentially reveal factors that influence injury risk, including the foot loading intensity (both high magnitude and short duration of loading) as well as development and remodeling in children (influenced by duration of loading and length of rest during toe walking) [9]. Previously, researchers have derived parameters using GRFs, such as peak forces, impulses, temporal events during the stance phase of gait to assess gait pathology [10]. Because toe walking is performed daily and frequently in this population, it is imperative to understand foot loading dynamics, slip and trip risk to intervene in cITW. A quantitative description of foot contact dynamics [11–14] and gait assessment may be helpful in (i) revealing severity of ITW, (ii) establishing norms among cITW, and (iii) devise intervention strategies.

It is well established that, during toe walking, increased plantarflexion can compromise gait stability and it is often associated with decreased walking speed and stride length [15,16]. To maintain an upright posture, one has to stabilize the center of mass (COM) over the base of support. Stabilizing the COM over a small base of support when advancing their body forward during walking is challenging for cITW who are described to produce a bouncy gait with higher energy expenditures. Along with inefficient gait, the toe walkers have sensory processing and integration issues [17,18]. Sensory integration is defined as the registration and modulation of input sensory signals (somatosensory, vision, and vestibular) to execute the movement. However, several studies have failed to demonstrate an enhanced sensory contribution to the muscle activity in toe walking children, and an alternative theory, which emphasizes altered central control as an adaptation to demands of muscle and joint mechanics, has been suggested [19–21]. It is not well known whether the toe walking observed among cITW is distinct as compared to the toe walking observed in healthy controls. It is also not known if angle of attack during foot initial contact (FIC) differs among cITW and will predispose them to falls. Given the dearth of evidence and inconsistent findings on toe walking among this particular population of ITW, this study's primary objective is to explore kinetic and gait differences during typical and toe walking and investigate how these influences fall risk. This study aims to examine how toe walking influences foot landing dynamics among cITW as compared to their healthy counter-parts and whether it predisposes them to trip risk and slip risk.

2. Materials and Methods

Ten cITW (five females, five males; age = 7.5 $\pm$ 2.3 years, weight = 60.8 $\pm$ 16.4 lbs, height = 49.6 $\pm$ 5.8 inches) and 10 healthy (five females, five males; age = 8.7 $\pm$ 3.4 years, weight = 69 $\pm$ 33.1 lbs, height = 51.2 $\pm$ 9.7 inches) children participated in this research. At recruitment, the diagnosed cITW participants were referred by a pediatric orthopedic surgeon and Orange county area physical therapist. All of the participants signed a written informed consent and the protocol was approved by the Children's Hospital of Orange County (CHOC) Institutional Review Board (IRB# 170870). CodaMotion 3-D Analysis System (Charnwood Dynamics Ltd., Leicestershire, UK) with four CODA optical sensors were used for data collection. The system captured the vertical, horizontal, and rotational movements by tracking the attached marker positions. The system consisted of infra-red light-emitting diode (LED) markers and drive boxes as marker devices, which were attached to bony anatomical landmarks at the skin. A cluster of four markers were placed at each segment (thigh, shank, upper arm, and pelvis). A total of 22 markers were placed bilaterally on the 5th metatarsal head, the base of the 5th metatarsal, with clusters placed on the shank, thigh, and pelvis. Clusters were used to mark virtual markers at the anterior superior iliac spine (ASIS), femoral head, lateral and medial femoral epicondyle, lateral tibial epicondyle, and medial and lateral malleoli. Codamotion ODIN software suite analyzed the data from sensor modules. The visibility of the markers was monitored in real-time during each walking trial. Functional joint centers, segment angles, and joint moments were computed using ODIN. The GRF data were collected using two forceplates model Bertec BP400600 (Bertec, Columbus, Ohio 43219). The GRF was filtered and normalized prior to evaluating the impact dynamics. For each trial evaluation, individual stance phases were parsed out, and outcome kinetic parameters were computed, as detailed below. The whole-body kinematics and GRFs were collected at 100 Hz and 1000 Hz, respectively, and then low-pass filtered at 6 Hz cut-off frequency (4th order, zero-lag Butterworth).

Procedures: the participants were asked to perform walking on a 10 m long walkway at their preferred pace. The walkway and surrounding area were well lit. The two forceplates were embedded at the center of the walkway. The participants were asked to walk in their natural or 'typical' way in which they usually walk at home and outside. The typical gait in cITW may be affected by the new testing environment, and children may consciously present best heel strikes during walking in clinicians' presence. One movement scientist with expertise in pediatrics physical therapy (PT) and two other PT's continuously interacted with the child participant and with parents to acclimatize participants to the new environment, such that the child could present typical walk during data collection. Two PT's stood on each side of the walkway with visual target and performance boards. The boards provided stars for every trial completion. The typical gait is different for cITW and healthy children. cITW usually perform toe-to-toe gait similar to toe walking, whereas healthy children perform a heel-to-toe gait. The second task was to perform toe walking, cITW performed this with higher plantarflexion angles than their typical walk. Each participant walked at least 10 trials of each walking type barefoot. The trial was repeated if the participants did not step at the center of the forceplate, or failed to perform the instructed kind of walk. The investigators visually checked for foot strike on forceplate and marked those trials as good. During data analysis, only three trials were randomly chosen from the trials that were marked as good for each walking type (typical and toe walking). The mean age and gender were balanced in both groups (ITW versus healthy controls).

Parameters from Vertical Ground Reaction Forces (GRF): vertical GRF was obtained when the participants walked over a forceplate that was embedded in the 10-m long walkway center. The vertical GRF was divided into a sequence of events (i) Foot initial Contact (FIC), (ii) Peak Loading Response (PLR), (iii) mid-stance (MS), (iv) peak push off (PPO), and (v) foot off (FO).

Loading rate is defined as the slope of vertical GRF from FIC to PLR. COM ascending rate is defined as the slope of vertical GRF from PLR to MS. COM descending rate is defined as the slope of vertical GRF from MS to PPO. Push off rate is defined as the slope of vertical GRF from PPO to FO. The times taken to reach these events are shown in Figure 1. Similarly, force impulses were computed as area under the GRF-time curve and defined as loading impulse, COM ascending impulse, COM descending impulse, and push-off impulse. The impulses were calculated, as shown by Equation (1) below. Where Vertical RF(t) is GRF at time t.

$$\text{Force Impulse} = \int_{t1}^{t2} \text{Vertical GRF}(t).dt \quad (1)$$

Joint angles were evaluated at the hip, knee, and ankle. Each segment was represented with three strategically placed markers to compute embedded vector basis (EVB) [22]. EVB was constructed using the Gram–Schmidt Orthogonalization method and embedded axes were aligned to be anatomically meaningful, as per ISB recommendations [22]. In the neutral position, joint angles are zero and they are quantified as segments reposition [23]. The foot segment angle was computed as the angle made by the line adjoining heel and toe markers with the horizontal axis (as shown in Figure 2).

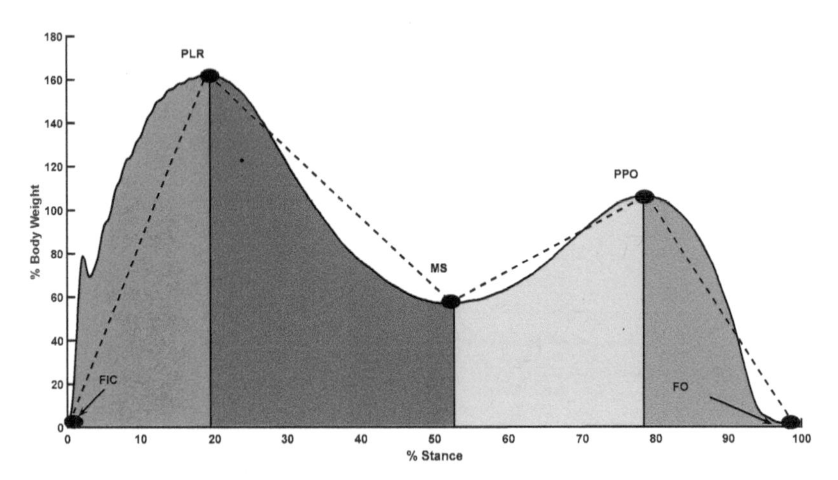

Figure 1. Stance vertical ground reaction force with events (i) foot initial contact (FIC), (ii) Peak Loading Response (PLR), (iii) mid-stance (MS), (iv) peak push off (PPO), and (v) foot off (FO). Slopes from FIC to PLR was defined as loading rate; PLR to MS as COM ascending rate; MS to PPO as COM descending rate; PPO to FO as Push off rate.

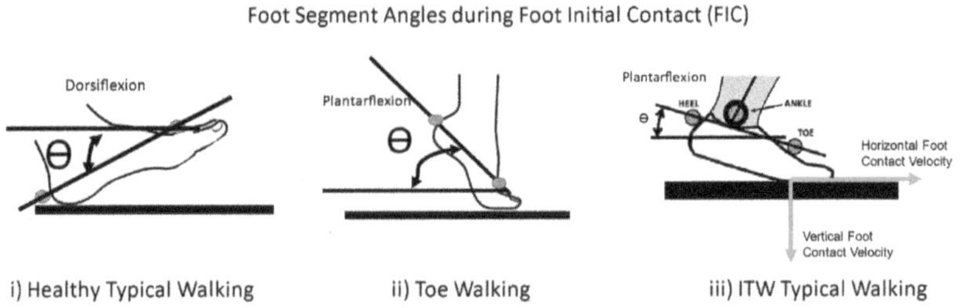

Foot Segment Angles during Foot Initial Contact (FIC)

Dorsiflexion

Plantarflexion

Plantarflexion

Horizontal Foot Contact Velocity

Vertical Foot Contact Velocity

i) Healthy Typical Walking

ii) Toe Walking

iii) ITW Typical Walking

Figure 2. Foot segment angles during foot initial contact for (**i**) healthy typical walking, (**ii**) toe walking, and (**iii**) Idiopathic Toe Walking (ITW) typical walking. Dorsiflexion angles are taken as positive and plantarflexion as negative.

Gait Assessments: foot contact was defined when the vertical force exceeded more than 7 N after the foot contacted the ground. In pilot trials, we placed heel and toe markers on lateral sides of the foot, such that foot initial contact determination (forceplate versus motion capture camera system) was consistently at about 7 N of vertical force. This could be due to signal noise from forceplate, which could not consistently detect force less than 7 N. The foot contact velocity was computed while utilizing the foot position marker at toe or heel, whichever impacts the ground surface during foot landing. The foot contact velocity was evaluated for horizontal and vertical directions through foot lowest marker displacement of 1/100 s before and after the foot contact phase of gait cycle using instantaneous foot velocity formula [24,25], as shown in Equation (2).

$$\text{Foot velocity} = \frac{(\text{Foot Marker Position}(i+1) - \text{Foot Marker Position}(i-1)}{2\Delta t} \quad (2)$$

Minimum Toe Clearance (MTC): it is the minimum vertical distance between the toe marker of the swing foot and the walking surface during swing. MTC is associated with trip-related falls during over ground walking [26–29].

Stride Time: it is the time taken from foot initial contact (FIC) to the next FIC of the same foot [30]. Stride Length: the distance that is covered during a stride time is stride length [30]. Transitional acceleration of COM is defined as the acceleration of COM during the foot initial contact [31], and it is represented in Equation (3) (Figure 3a).

$$\text{Transitional COM Acceleration} = \frac{(\text{COM Velocity}(\text{i}+1) - \text{COM Velocity}(\text{i}-1))}{2\Delta\text{t}} \quad (3)$$

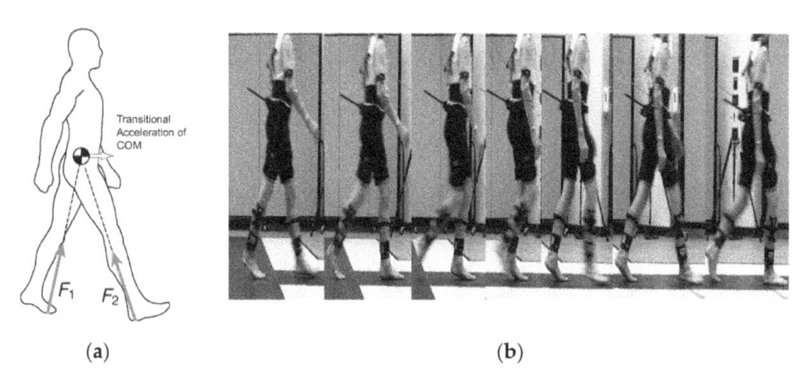

Figure 3. (**a**) Transitional acceleration of center of mass (COM) during walking (**b**) typical walking in cITW participant.

Mixed Factor MANOVA model analysis was conducted while using JMP Software (JMP 15 Pro, SAS Institute Inc., Cary, NC, USA), where the groups and walking type were fixed with subjects as random effects. The significance was set at $p = 0.05$. Post Hoc analysis was done using Tukey's HSD. We investigated multiple continuous dependent variables, and MANOVA bundles them together into a weighted linear combination. MANOVA will also compare if the combination differs by the different groups (typical, ITW) and levels of the independent variables (toe walking, typical walking). The model was tested for multicollinearity, normality, and homogeneity of variance. MANOVA was selected, since it has a greater statistical power than regular ANOVA. It can also limit the joint error rate as joint probability of rejecting a true null hypothesis increases with each additional test.

3. Results

3.1. Kinetic Data Analysis

There was no significant difference between groups (ITW versus healthy controls) across variables (i) loading rate, (ii) COM ascending rate, and (iii) COM descending rate. However, significant interaction effects were found between groups for push-off rate ($p < 0.01$) (Figure 3b). ITW were found to have significantly higher push-off rates during typical walking and significantly lower push off rate during toe walking when compared to healthy counterparts (Figure 4).

Similar results were found for force impulses during vertical GRF. No significant differences were observed for loading impulse, COM ascending impulse, and COM descending impulse, but interaction effects were found between groups and walking type for push-off impulse ($p < 0.01$). However, rates and force impulses for loading, COM ascending, COM descending, and push off were significantly different for the two walking types (typical versus toe walking) when combining all participants from both groups. The ankle, knee, and hip angles during stance events in cITW and controls have been reported for toe walking and typical gait (Table 1).

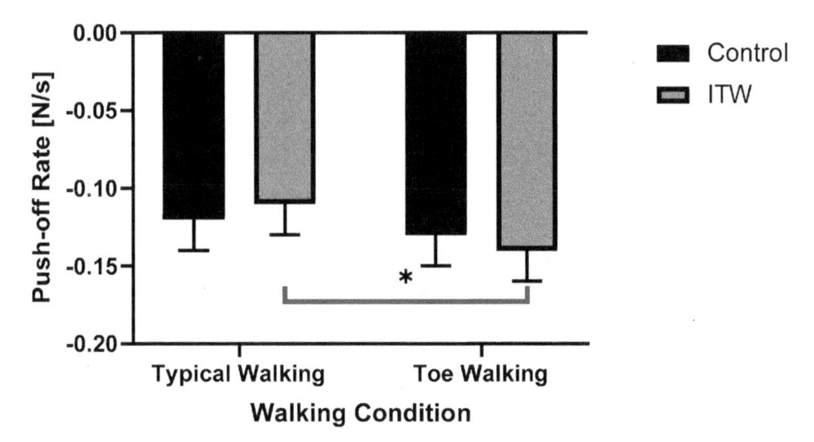

Figure 4. Push-off rate among ITW and Controls during typical and toe walking.

Table 1. Foot segment angle at FIC and FO and joint angles at loading, midstance, and push-off among ITW and controls. Here significant differences are represented by * ($p < 0.05$).

	Control		ITW	
Angles [Degrees]	**Toe Walking**	**Typical Walking**	**Toe Walking**	**Typical Walking**
Foot angle at FIC	−26.0 ± 17.1	1.6 ± 23.8	−29.1 ± 17.5	−16.3 ± 24.1
Foot angle at Foot Off (FO)	−43.2 ± 36.0	−41.1 ± 37.8	−47.2 ± 35.0	−34.0 ± 35.2
Ankle angle at Loading	−19.2 ± 16.9	−9.1 ± 13.4	−24.5 ± 16.6	−15.6 ± 12.7
Ankle angle at Midstance	−16.4 ± 8.7	3.7 ± 6.2	−22.8 ± 8.0	−6.2 ± 10.9
Ankle angle at Push−off	−25.8 ± 12.0	4.6 ± 8.8	−27.7 ± 9.1	−4.0 ± 11.5
Knee angle at Loading	25.2 ± 12.8	32.0 ± 14.2	25.5 ± 9.7	31.9 ± 16.4
Knee angle at Midstance	28.8 ± 23.0	30.2 ± 23.9	30.1 ± 23.3	38.5 ± 28.0
Knee angle at Push−off *	6.6 ± 13.0	4.1 ± 7.8	6.8 ± 8.9	11.1 ± 9.8
Hip angle at Loading	23.0 ± 36.6	24.7 ± 20.3	26.4 ± 22.9	25.2 ± 26.2
Hip angle at Midstance	19.3 ± 41.5	24.9 ± 16.0	28.9 ± 34.9	33.1 ± 20.3
Hip angle at Push−off	14.1 ± 39.4	14.1 ± 22.7	19.2 ± 39.9	28.2 ± 23.8

The time to reach mid-stance from foot initial contact was found to be significantly longer for toe walking when compared to typical walking for both groups ($p = 0.0001$). We found the time taken from push-off to foot off was significantly longer among ITW during their typical walking than toe walking ($p = 0.002$). We found that the ITW group produced significantly higher joint angles at the knee during push-off phase of typical walking ($p = 0.03$) as compared to healthy counterparts (Figure 5). Foot segment angles were significantly different for controls during foot initial contact ($p = 0.04$) (Figure 6). It was found that the foot dorsiflexed during FIC when typical walking and plantarflexed during FIC during toe walking. The joint angles at ankle during midstance were found to be significantly lower among ITW group as compared to the controls ($p = 0.006$).

We also found that during toe walking, joint angles at loading, mid-stance, and push-off were found to be significantly lower than typical walking among both groups ($p = 0.0005$).

3.2. *Gait Assessments*

The interaction effects were found to be significant ($p < 0.001$) for stride length between walking type (toe walking versus typical), and groups (ITW versus controls). Tukey's HSD revealed that controls produced longer strides during typical walking. Contrastingly cITW made longer strides during toe walking. Similarly, we found that the stride times were shorter during toe walking among both groups.

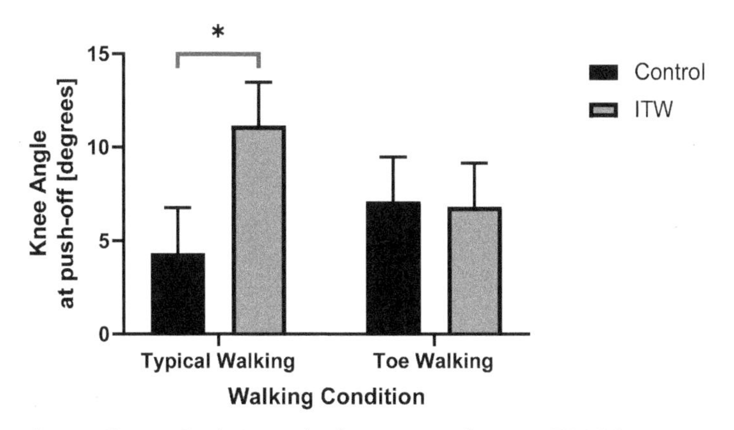

Figure 5. Knee angles during push-off among controls versus cITW. Where * represents significant difference with $p < 0.05$.

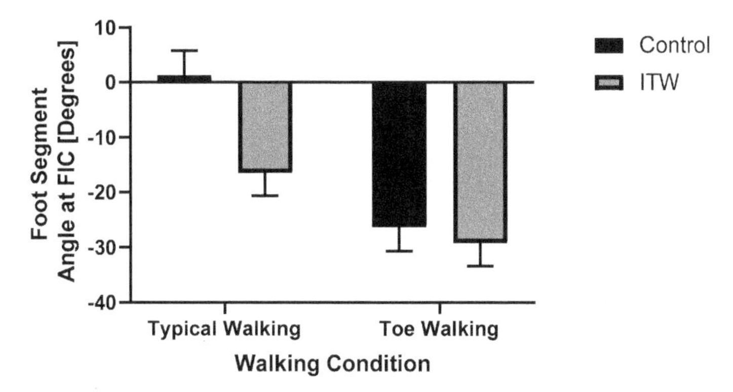

Figure 6. Foot segment angle at foot initial contact, dorsiflexion (positive), and plantarflexion (negative).

We found significant interaction effects ($p = 0.01$) for single stance time (SST). We found that cITW had longer SST during toe walking when compared to typical walking (Figure 7). Toe walking resulted in increased step width as compared to typical gait for both groups ($p = 0.0004$).

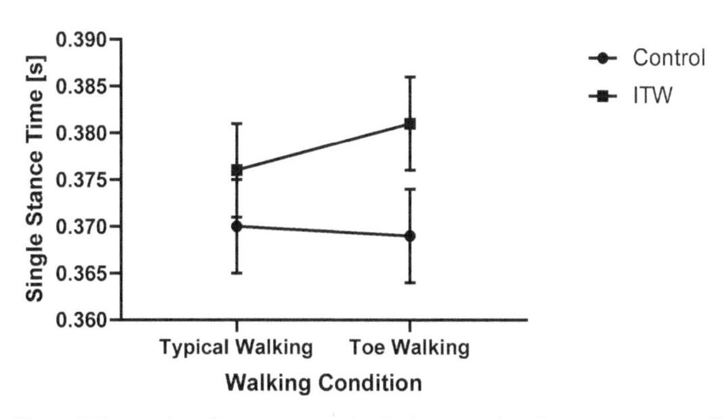

Figure 7. Interaction effects were seen in single stance time for group versus walking type.

Toe clearance significantly decreased among ITW during typical gait when compared to toe walking ($p = 0.005$) (Figure 8).

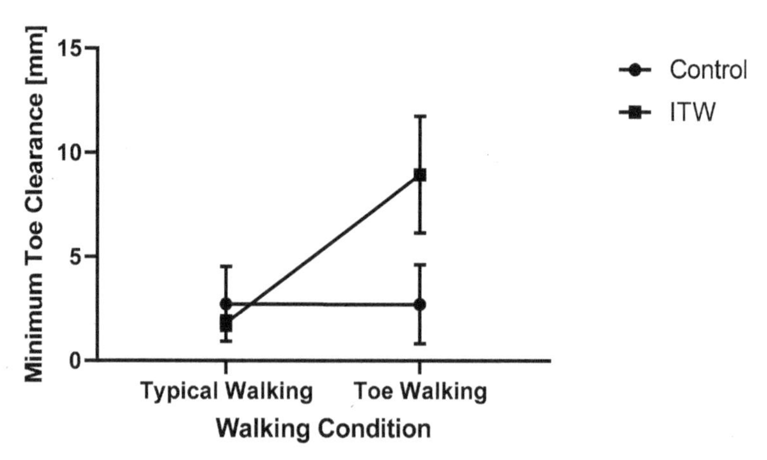

Figure 8. Interaction effects were seen in minimum toe clearance among groups and walking type.

Vertical foot contact velocity was significantly higher during toe walking among both of the groups ($p = 0.0004$) as compared to typical gait. Vertical foot contact velocity was the lowest among controls during typical gait. Horizontal foot contact velocity was found to be significantly higher during toe walking than typical walking among controls ($p = 0.0006$) (Figure 9).

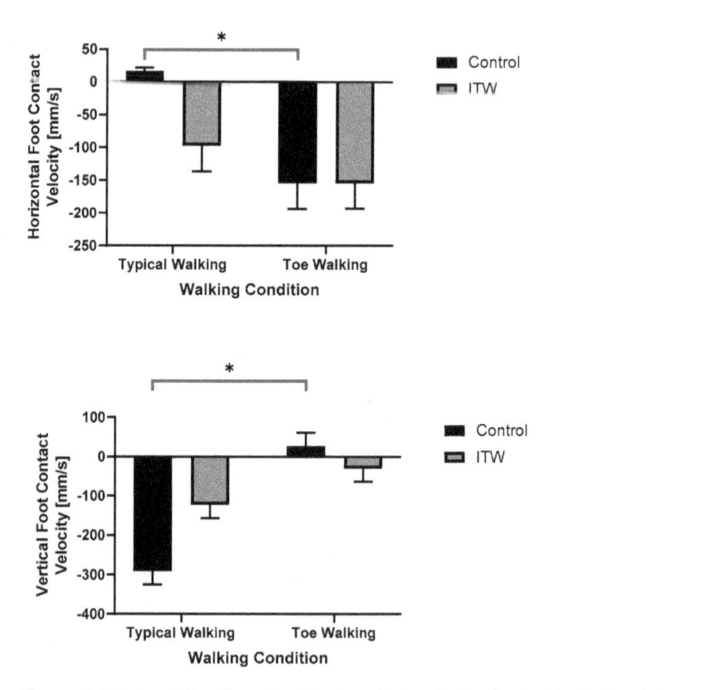

Figure 9. Horizontal and vertical foot contact velocity during typical and toe walking. Where * represents significant difference with $p < 0.05$.

Transitional Acceleration of COM was found lower among ITW during typical walking, but it was lower among the controls during toe walking. Table 2 reports all of these gait parameters for both the cITW and control group. In addition, mean joint angles during stance are reported for push off, swing, and FIC events shown in Table 3.

Table 2. Gait parameters associated with ITW and control. Here significant differences are represented by * ($p < 0.05$).

	Control		ITW	
	Toe Walking	Typical Walking	Toe Walking	Typical Walking
Stride Length * [mm]	921.4 ± 197.5	1066.0 ± 237.1	980.5 ± 169.3	911.2 ± 145.1
Stride Time [s]	0.8 ± 0.1	0.9 ± 0.1	0.8 ± 0.07	0.9 ± 0.1
Single Stance Duration [s]	0.3 ± 0.03	0.3 ± 0.01	0.3 ± 0.01	0.3 ± 0.03
Minimum Toe Clearance [mm]	2.7 ± 10.5	2.7 ± 11.1	8.9 ± 17.1	0.3 ± 13.1
Step Width [mm]	147.0 ± 38.9	133.6 ± 28.6	167.3 ± 41.3	145.2 ± 47.4
Horizontal Foot Contact Velocity [mm/s]	−154.3 ± 316.4	16.7 ± 176.7	−47.7 ± 220.0	−97.4 ± 231.4
Vertical Foot Contact Velocity * [mm/s]	27.3 ± 172.1	−291.2 ± 360.9	−29.3 ± 108.1	−123.1 ± 211.0
Transitional Acceleration of COM * [mm/s^2]	−288.0 ± 4771.5	782.94 ± 2631.8	1284.0 ± 3636.5	99.964 ± 2366.8

Table 3. Mean ± SD of Joint angles during push-off, swing and FIC for ankle, knee and hip for ITW and control with different walking types.

		Toe Walking			Typical Walking		
		Push-Off	Swing	FIC	Push-Off	Swing	FIC
Control [Degrees]	Ankle	−26.8 ± 12.4	−34.2 ± 8.0	−27.6 ± 10.3	1.8 ± 5.9	−15.4 ± 6.4	0.2 ± 5.5
	Knee	5.1 ± 9.8	25.6 ± 6.4	4.4 ± 8.7	1.5 ± 7.2	33.5 ± 6.6	1.7 ± 7.4
	Hip	38.0 ± 14.5	3.0 ± 12.9	36.3 ± 13.6	37.6 ± 12.8	2.2 ± 10.7	37.6 ± 11.3
ITW [Degrees]	Ankle	−34.6 ± 10.8	−39.7 ± 10.3	−33.5 ± 9.8	−9.9 ± 7.1	−19.1 ± 9.8	−8.7 ± 6.8
	Knee	1.4 ± 8.4	22.1 ± 5.7	1.8 ± 7.5	0.8 ± 5.0	32.2 ± 6.0	1.8 ± 5.1
	Hip	41.3 ± 15.2	4.5 ± 11.0	42.7 ± 13.8	38.7 ± 11.8	8.7 ± 12.2	40.0 ± 11.7

4. Discussion

Our major findings reveal that cITW are more prone to falls due to (i) lower toe clearance (increased trip risk), (ii) high horizontal heel velocity along with reduced transitional acceleration of COM (slip initiation risk), and (iii) reduced stability when stiffening during stance. We also found cITW typical walking to be inherently inefficient due to several reasons, such as (i) significantly higher push-off impulses, (ii) more knee flexion angles during stance, (iii) high vertical heel velocity, and (iv) already plantarflexed ankle fail to produce force generation capacity during push-off. These results have several broader impacts, for example, (i) foot segment angles and peak-push of impulses could possibly reveal critical insights into severity of ITW, (ii) since no previous study has established norms for foot contact dynamics among cITW population this study will serve as background work, (iii) new interventions, such as providing haptic feedback during toe walking [32] and identifying toe walking utilizing artificial intelligence [33], will help to develop novel interventions.

Toe walking may be associated with several other disorders and diagnoses, such as cerebral palsy (CP), muscular dystrophy, autism, myopathy, mental retardation, childhood schizophrenia, and muscular dystrophy [1,34,35]. Some researchers claim that ITW children do not have neurological signs [34], but only clinical signs of limited active dorsiflexion during gait. Others claim that ITW may be due to unknown deficits in the central nervous system or a neuropathic process as in muscle properties [36]. ITW children have been reported to have delayed the corticospinal tract [35]. Idiopathic toe walking is commonly diagnosed in pediatric orthopedic clinics as benign and it is often not informed to parents as a significant concern. If the complication gets aggravated with injuries, treatments, such as botox, casting, or ankle-foot orthotics (AFO), or even orthopedic surgery, is often recommended. Scientific knowledge lacks an objective assessment of ITW foot contact dynamics and how these influence slip and trip risk during walking as compared to age-matched healthy counterparts. In this study, we investigated ITW gait using kinetics and gait kinematics when walking in two different styles: (i) their usual or typical walking style and (ii) toe walking. Some advantages of using GRF in toe walking analysis include ease of use, non-invasive, portable forceplates, and they can be easily installed in clinical walking environments. The assessment of gait characteristics and risk of falls among cITW is challenging, since children can alter their gait while under observation in clinical laboratory. This makes gait analysis among ITW difficult with gait and fall risk underdiagnosed and underappreciated. To our knowledge, this is the first study investigating typical and toe walking differences among ITW and the age matched control population. The major findings are adaptations of cITW during push-off by producing significantly higher push-off rates and force impulses. They are also found to exhibit significantly higher joint angles at the knee level during the push-off. This adaptation at the knee joint through increased flexion angles during typical walking could be an extra burden on cITW and induce muscle fatigue and increase the risk of injuries.

Earlier researchers have used a kinematic analysis of ankle range of motion to differentiate ITW from CP [16,37–39]. We found that both ITW and control groups demonstrated significantly lower joint angles at loading, mid-stance, and push-off during toe walking (Table 1), suggesting rigidity at the lower extremity. The stiffening behavior and freezing the degree of freedom at the lower extremity joints could jeopardize gait stability and increase the chances of severe falls and injuries [40,41]. It was also found that foot segment angles at FIC were in the position of dorsiflexion for control typical walking, whereas it was at plantarflexion angle for cITW similar to toe walking (Figure 6). The magnitude of plantarflexion angles during FIC could serve as a score of ITW severity.

We also found that stride length was significantly longer during typical walking among both groups and shorter during toe walking. The reduced stride length indicates that toe walking is more restrictive with a limited degree of freedom to both groups and it will redistribute plantar foot pressures [42] to maintain COM over a smaller base of support. The single-limb stance time of gait is important, since, during this time, the foot is on the ground supporting the gravitational load of the whole body and propelling the COM forward, i.e., acting against the inertial and frictional load. A wide variety of force receptors are activated during stance, including cutaneous receptor, high threshold force receptor, and spindle from ankle joint muscles [43–45], to provide force feedback through afferent pathways [46]. The increased stance durations among cITW could adapt to acquire more proprioceptive and force feedback information to maintain stability compromising minimum plantar contact area with the ground. This compensation for stability is partially accommodated with increased step width, as found in our study. Although cITW seem to be exhibit coordinated walking, but their plantar weight-bearing is at the forefront of the foot, with plantarflexion ranging from 2.7 to 28.3 degrees during typical walking (Table 1). Ankle plantarflexion strength is primarily a function of moment arm from ankle joint to the ground reaction force line, acting at the center of pressure of the foot. During typical walking among the ITW group, the requirement for ankle plantarflexion is greatest in push-off. However, due to the already plantarflexed ankle, the force-generating capacity of ankle muscles reduces due to the limited range available for ankle plantarflexion. The neuromuscular demand on plantar flexors is greater for cITW [47–50]. These neuromuscular demands increase with an increase in moment arm during typical waling in cITW [51].

We also found that cITW had significantly lower toe clearance values during typical walking. A lower toe clearance has been associated with trip-related stumbles [52], and it imposes the highest risk of unintentional contact with obstacles or the ground [53]. This finding is important, since no previous study has reported trip risk among cITW. Along with trip risk, we evaluated slip initiation risk through foot contact velocity and transitional acceleration of COM. The horizontal foot contact velocity is reduced in healthy adults through the activation of the hamstring [25], but this stabilizing reduction in velocity was not observed in the ITW population (Table 2 and Figure 9). Thus, high horizontal heel contact velocity increases the slip initiation risk similarly to older adults. In addition, cITW are found to take a significantly longer time to reach mid-stance after foot initial contact during typical walking. This may have attributed to the significantly lower transitional acceleration of COM in ITW population. Transitional acceleration of COM has been reported to influence slip initiation (by modulating friction demand) [54,55]. The fall risk increases with the reduced acceleration of COM during walking. A repetitive high vertical foot contact velocity could increase the risk of injury due to the high ground impact.

We found that foot segment angles were significantly lower for ITW than controls (1.6° dorsiflexion as compared to 16.3° plantarflexion). This was attributed to higher horizontal foot contact velocity among cITW. Researchers have previously established a relationship with horizontal foot contact velocity and hamstring activation rate, ultimately leading to slip-induced fall accidents [25]. It is known that older adults have higher foot contact velocity when compared to younger adults due to slower hamstring activation rate, thereby modulating friction demand at the foot-floor interface and ultimately leading to increased likelihood of slip induced falls [25,31]. One potential limitation of this study is to acclimatize child participants to produce typical gait. However, the experiments included trained PT's, who continuously encouraged participants to maintain their typical gait by encouraging them to look forward at the target while walking and incentivizing through drawing stars once completing a walking trial.

5. Conclusions

Overall, this research has broader impacts in understanding fall risk and developing future novel personalized interventions for cITW using wearable sensors [32] and artificial intelligence [33]. This study will help to interpret gait characterization of ITW gait patterns, which would allow us to delineate using deviations that originate from ITW's typical walking versus induced toe-walking, both requiring different nervous control for compensatory adaptations. These adaptations are difficult to visualize by the naked eye, since subtle mechanical output during a movement in the multijointed human biomechanical system affects the whole lower extremity due to mechanical coupling. As per our knowledge, this is the first study looking into slip and trip risk variables that have considerable implications for clinicians and movement scientists in classifying the severity of toe walking and designing novel intervention tools for ITW.

Author Contributions: Conceptualization, R.S., R.B. and M.G.-B.; methodology, M.S., M.G.; software, M.S. and R.B.; validation, R.S., M.S., R.B., M.G.-B. and M.G.; formal analysis, R.B.; investigation, R.S., R.B., and M.G.-B.; resources, M.G.-B.; data curation, M.S.; writing—original draft preparation, R.S.; writing—review and editing, L.B., V.M., M.T., A.A.; visualization, R.S.; supervision, M.G.-B.; project administration, R.S., M.G.-B.; funding acquisition, M.G.-B. All authors have read and agreed to the published version of the manuscript.

Funding: This research was funded by Kay Family Foundation and CHOC-Transformational Philanthropic Venture Funding Program and The APC was funded by CHOC.

Institutional Review Board Statement: The study was conducted according to the guidelines of the Declaration of Helsinki, and approved by the Institutional Review Board (or Ethics Committee) of CHOC (IRB#170870 protocol code and 08/2017 as date of approval).

Informed Consent Statement: Informed consent was obtained from all subjects involved in the study. Written informed consent has been obtained from the patient(s) to publish this paper.

Acknowledgments: We are thankful to Christopher Hoang, and DPT students during data collection.

Conflicts of Interest: The authors declare no conflict of interest.

References

1. Sobel, E.; Caselli, M.; Velez, Z. Effect of persistent toe walking on ankle equinus. Analysis of 60 idiopathic toe walkers. *J. Am. Podiatr. Med. Assoc.* **1997**, *87*, 17–22. [CrossRef]
2. Sutherland, D.H.; Olshen, R.; Cooper, L.; Woo, S.L. The development of mature gait. *J. Bone Jt. Surg. Am.* **1980**, *62*, 336–353. [CrossRef]
3. Fox, A.; Deakin, S.; Pettigrew, G.; Paton, R. Serial casting in the treatment of idiopathic toe-walkers and review of the literature. *Acta Orthop. Belg.* **2006**, *72*, 722–730.
4. Hirsch, G.; Wagner, B. The natural history of idiopathic toe-walking: A long-term follow-up of fourteen conservatively treated children. *Acta Paediatr.* **2004**, *93*, 196–199. [CrossRef]
5. Tabrizi, P.; McIntyre, W.M.J.; Quesnel, M.B.; Howard, A.W. Limited dorsiflexion predisposes to injuries of the ankle in children. *J. Bone Jt. Surg. Br.* **2000**, *82*, 1103–1106. [CrossRef]
6. Tardieu, C.; Lespargot, A.; Tabary, C.; Bret, M.D. Toe-walking in children with cerebral palsy: Contributions of contracture and excessive contraction of triceps surae muscle. *Phys. Ther.* **1989**, *69*, 656–662. [CrossRef] [PubMed]
7. Gross, R.; Leboeuf, F.; Hardouin, J.B.; Perrouin-Verbe, B.; Brochard, S.; Rémy-Néris, O. Does muscle coactivation influence joint excursions during gait in children with and without hemiplegic cerebral palsy? Relationship between muscle coactivation and joint kinematics. *Clin. Biomech.* **2015**, *30*, 1088–1093. [CrossRef]
8. Kedem, P.; Scher, D.M. Foot deformities in children with cerebral palsy. *Curr. Opin. Pediatr.* **2015**, *27*, 67–74. [CrossRef]
9. Edwards, W.B. Modeling overuse injuries in sport as a mechanical fatigue phenomenon. *Exerc. Sport Sci. Rev.* **2018**, *46*, 224–231. [CrossRef]
10. Chao, E.; Laughman, R.; Schneider, E.; Stauffer, R. Normative data of knee joint motion and ground reaction forces in adult level walking. *J. Biomech.* **1983**, *16*, 219–233. [CrossRef]
11. Rodda, J.M.; Graham, H.K.; Carson, L.; Galea, M.P.; Wolfe, R. Sagittal gait patterns in spastic diplegia. *J. Bone Jt. Surg. Br.* **2004**, *86*, 251–258. [CrossRef]
12. Winters, T.F., Jr.; Gage, J.R.; Hicks, R. Gait patterns in spastic hemiplegia in children and young adults. *J. Bone Jt. Surg. Am.* **1987**, *69*, 437–441.
13. Lin, C.-J.; Guo, L.-Y.; Su, F.-C.; Chou, Y.-L.; Cherng, R.-J. Common abnormal kinetic patterns of the knee in gait in spastic diplegia of cerebral palsy. *Gait Posture* **2000**, *11*, 224–232. [CrossRef]
14. Armand, S.; Watelain, E.; Mercier, M.; Lensel, G.; Lepoutre, F.-X. Identification and classification of toe-walkers based on ankle kinematics, using a data-mining method. *Gait Posture* **2006**, *23*, 240–248. [CrossRef]
15. Davids, J.R.; Foti, T.; Dabelstein, J.; Bagley, A. Voluntary (normal) versus obligatory (cerebral palsy) toe-walking in children: A kinematic, kinetic, and electromyographic analysis. *J. Pediatr. Orthop.* **1999**, *19*, 461–469. [CrossRef] [PubMed]
16. Hicks, R.; Durinick, N.; Gage, J.R. Differentiation of idiopathic toe-walking and cerebral palsy. *J. Pediatr. Orthop.* **1988**, *8*, 160–163. [CrossRef]
17. Chu, V.; Anderson, L. Sensory-processing differences in children with idiopathic toe walking (ITW). *Am. J. Occup. Ther.* **2020**, *74*, 7411505130. [CrossRef]
18. Williams, C.M.; Tinley, P.; Curtin, M. Idiopathic toe walking and sensory processing dysfunction. *J. Foot Ankle Res.* **2010**, *3*, 16. [CrossRef]
19. Berger, W.; Quintern, J.; Dietz, V. Pathophysiology of gait in children with cerebral palsy. *Electroencephalogr. Clin. Neurophysiol.* **1982**, *53*, 538–548. [CrossRef]
20. Gough, M.; Shortland, A.P. Could muscle deformity in children with spastic cerebral palsy be related to an impairment of muscle growth and altered adaptation? *Dev. Med. Child Neurol.* **2012**, *54*, 495–499. [CrossRef]
21. Willerslev-Olsen, M.; Andersen, J.B.; Sinkjaer, T.; Nielsen, J.B. Sensory feedback to ankle plantar flexors is not exaggerated during gait in spastic hemiplegic children with cerebral palsy. *J. Neurophysiol.* **2014**, *111*, 746–754. [CrossRef]
22. Wu, G.; Siegler, S.; Allard, P.; Kirtley, C.; Leardini, A.; Rosenbaum, D.; Whittle, M.; D'Lima, D.D.; Cristofolini, L.; Witte, H.; et al. ISB recommendation on definitions of joint coordinate system of various joints for the reporting of human joint motion—part I: Ankle, hip, and spine. *J. Biomech.* **2002**, *35*, 543–548. [CrossRef]
23. Grood, E.S.; Suntay, W.J. A joint coordinate system for the clinical description of three-dimensional motions: Application to the knee. *J. Biomech. Eng.* **1983**, *105*, 136–144. [CrossRef] [PubMed]
24. Winter, D.A. *Biomechanics and Motor Control of Human Movement*, 4th ed.; Wiley: Hoboken, NJ, USA, 2009.
25. Lockhart, T.E.; Kim, S. Relationship between hamstring activation rate and heel contact velocity: Factors influencing age-related slip-induced falls. *Gait Posture* **2006**, *24*, 23–34. [CrossRef]
26. Barrett, R.; Mills, P.; Begg, R. A systematic review of the effect of ageing and falls history on minimum foot clearance characteristics during level walking. *Gait Posture* **2010**, *32*, 429–435. [CrossRef]
27. Khandoker, A.H.; Lynch, K.; Karmakar, C.K.; Begg, R.K.; Palaniswami, M. Regulation of minimum toe clearance variability in the young and elderly during walking on sloped surfaces. In Proceedings of the 29th Annual International Conference of the IEEE Engineering in Medicine and Biology Society, Lyon, France, 23–26 August 2007; pp. 4887–4890.
28. Murray, M.P.; Clarkson, B.H. The vertical pathways of the foot during level walking. I. Range of variability in normal men. *Phys. Ther.* **1966**, *46*, 585–589. [CrossRef]

29. Nagano, H.; Begg, R.; Sparrow, W.A. Computation method for available response time due to tripping at minimum foot clearance. In Proceedings of the 35th Annual International Conference of the IEEE Engineering in Medicine and Biology Society (EMBC), Osaka, Japan, 3–7 July 2013; pp. 4899–4902. [CrossRef]
30. Hollman, J.H.; McDade, E.M.; Petersen, R.C. Normative spatiotemporal gait parameters in older adults. *Gait Posture* **2011**, *34*, 111–118. [CrossRef] [PubMed]
31. Lockhart, T.E.; Woldstad, J.C.; Smith, J.L. Effects of age-related gait changes on the biomechanics of slips and falls. *Ergonomics* **2003**, *46*, 1136–1160. [CrossRef] [PubMed]
32. Pollind, M.; Soangra, R.; Grant-Beuttler, M.; Aminian, A. Customized wearable sensor-based insoles for gait re-training in idiopathic toe walkers. *Biomed. Sci. Instrum.* **2019**, *55*, 192–198.
33. Kim, S.; Soangra, R.; Grant-Beuttler, M.; Aminian, A. Wearable sensor-based gait classification in idiopathic toe walking adolescents. *Biomed. Sci. Instrum.* **2019**, *55*, 178–185.
34. Sala, D.A.; Shulman, L.H.; Kennedy, R.F.; Grant, A.D.; Chu, M.L. Idiopathic toe-walking: A review. *Dev. Med. Child. Neurol.* **1999**, *41*, 846–848. [CrossRef] [PubMed]
35. A Caselli, M.; Rzonca, E.C.; Lue, B.Y. Habitual toe-walking: Evaluation and approach to treatment. *Clin. Podiatr. Med. Surg.* **1988**, *5*, 547–559.
36. Eastwood, D.M.; Dennett, X.; Shield, L.K.; Dickens, D.R.V. Muscle abnormalities in idiopathic toe-walkers. *J. Pediatr. Orthop. B* **1997**, *6*, 215–218. [CrossRef]
37. Rose, J.; Martin, J.G.; Torburn, L.; Rinsky, L.A.; Gamble, J.G. Electromyographic differentiation of diplegic cerebral palsy from idiopathic toe walking: Involuntary coactivation of the quadriceps and gastrocnemius. *J. Pediatr. Orthop.* **1999**, *19*, 677–682. [CrossRef]
38. Policy, J.F.; Torburn, L.; Rinsky, L.A.; Rose, J. Electromyographic test to differentiate mild diplegic cerebral palsy and idiopathic toe-walking. *J. Pediatr. Orthop.* **2001**, *21*, 784–789. [CrossRef] [PubMed]
39. Kelly, I.P.; Jenkinson, A.; Stephens, M.; O'Brien, T. The kinematic patterns of toe-walkers. *J. Pediatr. Orthop.* **1997**, *17*, 478–480. [CrossRef]
40. Choi, H.S.; Baek, Y.S. Effects of the degree of freedom and assistance characteristics of powered ankle-foot orthoses on gait stability. *PLoS ONE* **2020**, *15*, e0242000. [CrossRef]
41. Chen, S.K.; Voaklander, D.; Perry, D.; Jones, C.A. Falls and fear of falling in older adults with total joint arthroplasty: A scoping review. *BMC Musculoskelet Disord.* **2019**, *20*, 1–8. [CrossRef]
42. Allet, L.; Ijzerman, H.; Meijer, K.; Willems, P.; Savelberg, H. The influence of stride-length on plantar foot-pressures and joint moments. *Gait Posture* **2011**, *34*, 300–306. [CrossRef]
43. Cleland, C.L.; Hayward, L.; Rymer, W.Z. Neural mechanisms underlying the clasp-knife reflex in the cat. II. Stretch-sensitive muscular-free nerve endings. *J. Neurophysiol.* **1990**, *64*, 1319–1330. [CrossRef]
44. Cleland, C.L.; Rymer, W.Z.; Edwards, F.R.; Gabrielli, B.; Roy, L.; Maller, J. Force-sensitive interneurons in the spinal cord of the cat. *Science* **1982**, *217*, 652–655. [CrossRef] [PubMed]
45. Rymer, W.Z.; Houk, J.C.; Crago, P.E. Mechanisms of the clasp-knife reflex studied in an animal model. *Exp. Brain Res.* **1979**, *37*, 93–113. [CrossRef] [PubMed]
46. Duysens, J.; Clarac, F.; Cruse, H. Load-regulating mechanisms in gait and posture: Comparative aspects. *Physiol. Rev.* **2000**, *80*, 83–133. [CrossRef] [PubMed]
47. Neptune, R.R.; Burnfield, J.M.; Mulroy, S.J. The neuromuscular demands of toe walking: A forward dynamics simulation analysis. *J. Biomech.* **2007**, *40*, 1293–1300. [CrossRef] [PubMed]
48. Gravel, D.; Richards, C.L.; Filion, M. Influence of contractile tension development on dynamic strength measurements of the plantarflexors in man. *J. Biomech.* **1988**, *21*, 89–96. [CrossRef]
49. Nistor, L.; Markhede, G.; Grimby, G. A technique for measurements of plantar flexion torque with the Cybex II dynamometer. *Scand. J. Rehabil. Med.* **1982**, *14*, 163–166.
50. Sale, D.; Quinlan, J.; Marsh, E.; McComas, A.J.; Bélanger, A.Y. Influence of joint position on ankle plantarflexion in humans. *J. Appl. Physiol.* **1982**, *52*, 1636–1642. [CrossRef]
51. Rugg, S.; Gregor, R.; Mandelbaum, B.; Chiu, L. In vivo moment arm calculations at the ankle using magnetic resonance imaging (MRI). *J. Biomech.* **1990**, *23*, 495–501. [CrossRef]
52. Rosenblatt, N.J.; Bauer, A.; Grabiner, M.D. Relating minimum toe clearance to prospective, self-reported, trip-related stumbles in the community. *Prosthetics Orthot. Int.* **2017**, *41*, 387–392. [CrossRef]
53. Killeen, T.; Easthope, C.S.; Demkó, L.; Filli, L.; Lőrincz, L.; Linnebank, M.; Curt, A.; Zörner, B.; Bolliger, M. Minimum toe clearance: Probing the neural control of locomotion. *Sci. Rep.* **2017**, *7*, 1922. [CrossRef]
54. Lockhart, T.E.; Woldstad, J.C.; Smith, J.L. Relationship between transitional acceleration of the whole body center-of-mass and friction demand characteristic during gait. In Proceedings of the Human Factors and Ergonomics Society Annual Meeting, Baltimore, MD, USA, 29 September–4 October 2002; SAGE Publications: Thousand Oaks, CA, USA, 2002; Volume 46, pp. 1186–1190.
55. Kim, S.; Lockhart, T.; Yoon, H.-Y. Relationship between age-related gait adaptations and required coefficient of friction. *Saf. Sci.* **2005**, *43*, 425–436. [CrossRef] [PubMed]

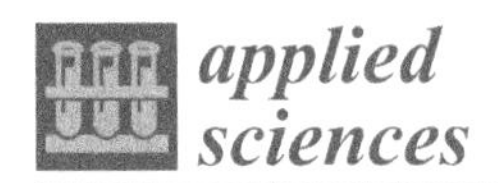

MDPI

Article

Postural Instability after Stepping on a Stair in Older Adults: A Pilot Study

Hyokeun Lee [1] and Kyungseok Byun [1,2,*]

1 Biomechanics Research Laboratory, Vector Biomechanics, Inc., Seoul 08506, Korea; leeh82@gmail.com
2 Department of Leisure & Sports, Kyungpook National University, Sangju 37224, Korea
* Correspondence: vbiomechanics@gmail.com; Tel.: +82-10-2876-3815

Abstract: This study aimed to examine how older adults (OA) control their postural stability after stepping on a stair in comparison to young adults (YA). Ten OA and 10 YA participated in this study. Participants ascended a single stair (15 cm high by 30 cm wide) which was secured atop one of the force plates. Ground reaction forces (GRFs) and center of pressure (COP) motion data were obtained from the force plate under the stair. After standing on the stair with both feet, GRFs and COP data for a 3 s duration were analyzed to assess postural variables, including time to stabilization (TTS), COP velocity (COPVEL), and COP sway area (COPSWAY). A significant difference in TTS in the anterior–posterior direction between OA and YA ($p = 0.032$) was observed, indicating that OA had difficulty stabilizing their body posture after the stair ascent compared to YA. For COP postural variables, no significant differences in COPVEL ($p = 0.455$) and COPSWAY ($p = 0.176$) were observed between OA and YA. Study findings indicate that older adults have less capacity to regain postural stability compared to young adults following a challenging dynamic movement.

Keywords: postural stability; older adults; stepping on a stair; time to stabilization

Citation: Lee, H.; Byun, K. Postural Instability after Stepping on a Stair in Older Adults: A Pilot Study. *Appl. Sci.* **2021**, *11*, 11885. https://doi.org/10.3390/app112411885

Academic Editor: Nyeonju Kang

Received: 28 October 2021
Accepted: 13 December 2021
Published: 14 December 2021

1. Introduction

Postural instability in older adults (OA) leads to impaired balance control when performing activities of daily living, potentially causing an increased risk and incidence of falls and a reduction of independence and quality of life [1]. Given that the biomechanical mechanisms of postural instability in OA have been well documented [2], the balance deficits of OA have been shown to manifest not only during static movements [3], but also during dynamic transitive movement in daily activities [4].

A stair ascent task is a functionally relevant motor task that significantly challenges the locomotor and postural control system. Biomechanically, stair ascent requires significant momentum, which is necessary for conjoint upward and forward body propulsion [5]. Indeed, stabilizing one's body posture following stair ascent is needed to offset the propulsive momentum generated by the whole body. Accordingly, individuals with strength deficits may be more impaired at controlling stability after a stair ascent task, exhibiting alterations in their strength compensation strategy. Indeed, it has been reported that individuals with muscular and neurologic deficits (e.g., osteoarthritis and stroke) are at a greater risk of having a stepping-related fall due to biomechanical and environmental constraints [6,7].

When comparing OA and YA (young adults), OA are at higher risk of loss of balance and falls during stair ascent in comparison to YA, in part due to muscular deficits. Specifically, muscle weakness in the elderly causes abnormal gait patterns and changes their gait biomechanics, particularly affecting gait velocity, and with less strength in their lower extremities leading to their greater incidence of falls [8,9]. Despite greater predicted possibilities that OA show balance problems and falls, studies have thus far focused less on motor control in dynamic activities, such as stepping up stairs, and even less on comparatively examining OA and YA.

Additionally, stair ascent is a complex task that is cognitively demanding compared to other simple tasks (e.g., sit-to-stand) [10], and age differences in cognitive abilities have been clearly shown [11]. A study proposed that significantly more attentional resources are required during stair ascent in OA than YA, while greater attentional resources are not required during simple tasks, such as standing [12]. It is also highlighted that cognitive decline is a common problem observed in the elderly [13]. Thus, stair ascent task assessments provide important insights into biomechanical abilities that cannot be captured through simple tasks for OA, while being sensitive to different cognitive abilities by age.

The purpose of the current study was to examine how stabilizing capabilities after stepping up stairs in OA faired in comparison to YA, hypothesizing that OA would take longer to stabilize their body posture and would have less ability to regain static plateau after the stepping performance. To find the exact time point at which one's postural sway is in plateau, we utilized the 'time to stabilization (TTS)' metric, which provides underlying information calculated based on overall information in a time series. It is useful and applicable when assessing dynamic balance capability.

2. Materials and Methods

2.1. Participants

Ten OA (Age: 71 ± 4.2 yr, height: 170.6 ± 5.4 cm, body mass: 73.2 ± 9.4 kg) and 10 YA (age: 27 ± 6 yr, height: 172.1 ± 7.4 cm, body mass: 72.5 ± 13.8 kg) participated in this study. All participants were asked to perform a cognition test (the mini-mental state examination, or MMSE) for screening purposes, and those who obtained a score of 23 or under were excluded from participating in the study. Participants had not had any musculoskeletal problems within the past six months and had not had any recent surgery. Informed consent was reviewed with each participant, and once all questions were answered and the documentation of consent was obtained, the experimental session began.

2.2. Experimental Protocol

Sixteen passive reflective markers were attached to the lower body in accordance with the instructions that accompanied the Helen Hays marker set, and kinematic data were collected using a 10-camera motion capture system (100 Hz, Qualisys, Gothenburg, Sweden). For the stair ascent trial, participants ascended a single stair (18 cm high by 40 cm wide), which was secured atop one of the force plates, barefoot. In response to a verbal signal of "ready", participants were asked to wait a moment and then begin the movement by stepping onto the stair with their dominant leg and maintain their stability (for at least 5 s) in a static position once both feet were atop the stair. Further, during the stepping task, participants were asked to fold their arms across their chest. The events of the stepping performance, including (1) the initial foot being raised from the ground, (2) the initial foot making contact with the stair, (3) the second foot being raised from the ground, and (4) the second foot making contact with the stair, were identified based on the ground reaction force data and the feet kinematic data. Ground reaction forces (GRFs) and moments were recorded using two force plates, one mounted on the laboratory floor and the other on the stair (300 Hz, Kistler, Winterthur, Swiss) (Figure 1). We measured GRFs and center of pressure (COP) motion along the anterior–posterior (AP) and mediolateral (ML) axes of motion for data analysis, and filtered GRF and COP data using a second-order Butterworth low-pass filter with a cutoff frequency of 5 Hz. GRFs and COP data were captured for a duration of 3 s after both feet were standing on the stair to assess the subjects' postural stabilization.

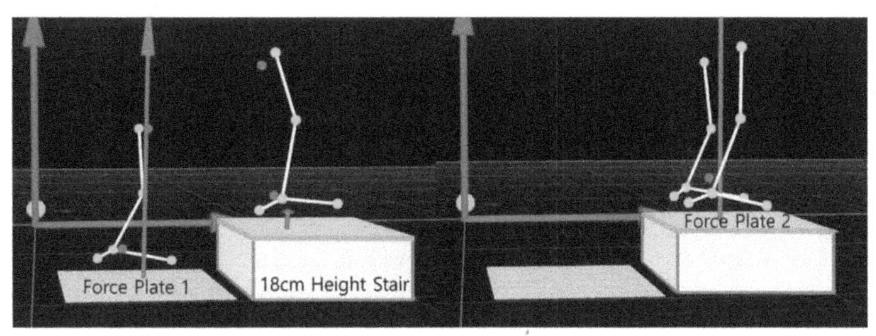

Figure 1. Experimental protocol of the stepping on a stair task with two force plates, one mounted on the laboratory floor (the first plate) and the other on the stair (the second plate).

2.3. Data Reduction and Processing

We obtained GRF and center of pressure (COP) motion data along the anterior–posterior (AP) and medial–lateral (ML) axes of motion for data analysis, and filtered the GRF and COP data using a second-order Butterworth low-pass filter with a cutoff frequency of 5 Hz. GRFs and COP data were measured for a duration of 3 s after both feet were standing on the stair (event four: when the second foot came into contact with the stair) to assess the subjects' postural stabilization.

Time to stabilization (TTS) scores for the AP and ML directions were separately calculated according to the ground reaction forces (x vector, AP; y vector, ML). As a sequential estimation, TTS incorporates an algorithm to calculate a cumulative average of the data points in a series by successively adding one point at a time [14]. This cumulative average value is sequentially compared with the overall series mean. When the value of the sequential average passes through a level that is within 0.25 SDs of the overall series mean, the individual series is considered to be at a plateau stage. The series consists of all data points within the first 3 s of both feet making contact with the stair (Figure 2).

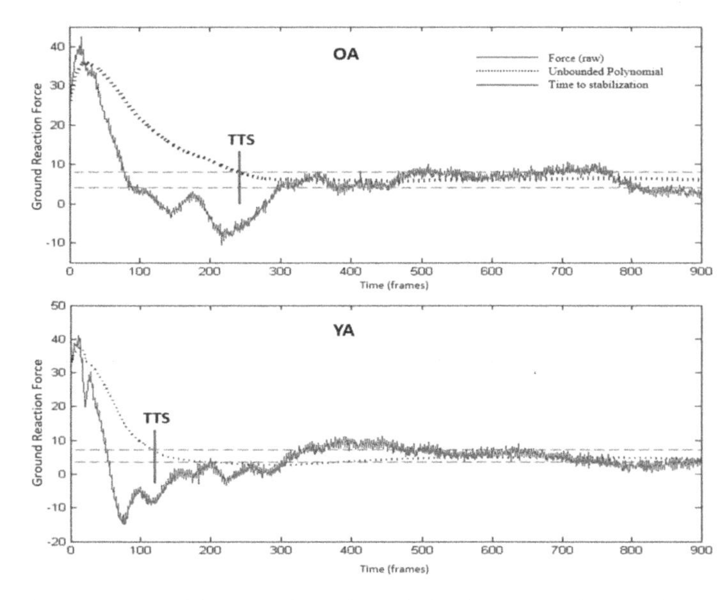

Figure 2. Time to stabilization in OA and YA calculated using ground reaction forces measure-ments.

For the traditional postural assessment, we also calculated COP velocity (COPVEL) and sway of 95% confidence ellipse (COPSWAY), which were calculated around the filtered COP motion along both the AP and ML axes (Figure 3). The details regarding the procedure to calculate COPVEL and the COPSWAY are described in previous literature [15,16].

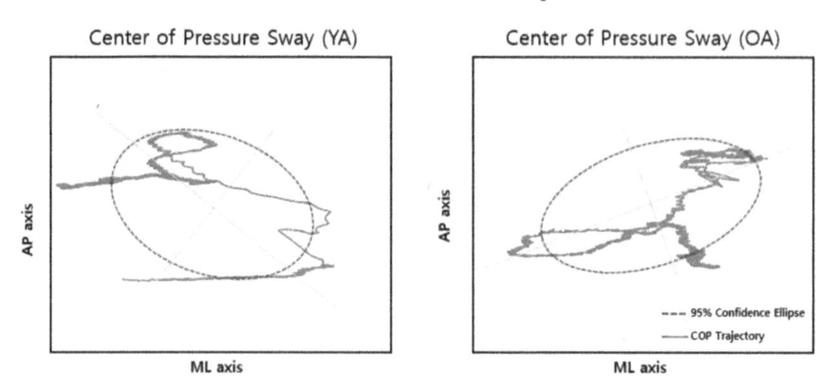

Figure 3. The center of pressure (COP) trajectories during posture stabilization after a stepping movement in OA and YA.

2.4. Statistical Analysis

Descriptive statistics for age, body mass, height, and MMSE were calculated for both groups. Independent *t*-tests were used to compare all dependent variables between OA and YA. Statistical analyses were performed using SPSS, and all levels of significance were set at $\alpha = 0.05$.

3. Results

A significant difference in TTS AP between OA and YA ($p = 0.032$) and a marginal but not statistical difference in TTS ML ($p = 0.141$) were observed, indicating that OA needed a longer time to stabilize their body posture after stair ascent compared to YA. For COP postural variables, no significant difference in COPVEL ($p = 0.455$) and COPSWAY ($p = 0.176$) were observed between OA and YA (Table 1).

Table 1. Mean, standard deviation, and *p*-value from *t*-tests for all dependent variables, including TTS AP, TTS ML, COPVEL, and COPSWAY. $p < 0.05$ for difference between OA and YA.

Variables	Older Adults (OA)	Young Adults (YA)	*p*-Value
Time to Stabilization (AP)	1.62 ± 0.15	1.26 ± 0.12	$p = 0.032$ *
Time to Stabilization (ML)	1.85 ± 0.21	1.82 ± 0.23	$p = 0.141$
COPVEL (cm/s)	0.84 ± 0.23	0.81 ± 0.25	$p = 0.455$
COPSWAY (CE95%, cm^2)	31.4 ± 12.1	0.81 ± 0.25	$p = 0.176$

* Significant difference between OA and YA at $p < 0.05$.

4. Discussion

There have been only a few studies using time to stabilization (TTS) to assess postural capacity in older adults (OA) or disease populations. A previous study utilized TTS to assess how stroke patients control their postural stability in response to unpredicted perturbation [17]. They reported that stroke patients who had intensive weighted training showed decreased TTS scores, indicating their improved capacity to stabilize their postural sway in the face of unpredicted perturbations. Bieryla and Madigan [18] further demonstrated that an improvement in one's postural stability as measured by TTS was observed more in older adults who had exercise training than those without training.

To our knowledge, this preliminary investigation is the first to assess the stabilization capacity of OA following a stepping movement, as measured by TTS. There have been a few studies that have compared spatiotemporal measures and the stabilizing strategies of OA and YA during stair ascent. One study reported that there were no significant group differences in stepping performance [19], while another study reported that OA show smaller separations between the center of mass and the center of pressure, which is indicative of different stepping strategies between groups [20]. However, no study examined the stabilization capacity after the stepping movement had been completed. By using TTS in this study, we tried to account for the deficits of stabilizing capacity in OA during a challenging dynamic movement. As hypothesized, OA exhibited a significantly longer time to stabilize their postural sway following stair ascent in comparison to YA. This finding indicated that OA may have less capacity to regain postural stability compared to YA following a challenging task, such as stepping on a stair. Given that a longer time for stabilization is highly correlated with a greater risk of falls [21], our TTS finding supports the observation that OA are at a greater risk of falls compared to YA. The finding of the current study could potentially provide a reliable and objective index for the evaluation of dynamic postural stability in OA.

However, we did not observe any significant differences between OA and YA in balance performance during posture stabilization after stepping on a stair when we assessed this using COP measures (e.g., COPVEL and COPSWAY). Conventionally, balance problems in OA have been identified by evaluating the COP motion [22]. For example, greater velocity or sway area during static movement has been considered to be one of the representative characteristics of postural control deficits in OA [23]. Biomechanically, however, dynamic movement, such as stair ascent, require a sufficient level of body momentum and co-contraction between COP and the body's center of mass to maintain postural stability when compensating for propulsive body momentum [24]. Unlike static standing, such dynamic movements are likely performed with greater variation because the majority of factors (e.g., force generation, cognition, and the environment itself) are consistently working as determining contributors to overall dynamic performance [25]. Therefore, it is difficult to account for postural capacity by using traditional COP measures, such as sway area or velocity, when biomechanically investigating dynamic balance.

There were limitations to the current pilot study. In a previous biomechanical study measuring TTS in athlete populations, it was reported that ankle joint stability, braces, and fatigue were closely related to TTS, indicating that ankle joint functions play a crucial role in dynamic balance and time to stabilization when experiencing an external perturbation [26]. Although previous studies investigated the balance recovery function using the TTS measure, which is consistent with our investigation, results from the current study should be interpreted with careful consideration. Particularly, unlike a previous study [27], subjects in our investigation were screened out when they had any musculoskeletal problems and fatigue. Therefore, we speculate that there might be other factors that affect TTS scores (e.g., muscle strength), which clearly differentiated the balance recovery functions between OA and YA.

5. Conclusions

The findings in this study will have the potential to give us a better understanding of how the elderly experience postural instability in daily life. More research is needed, however, to confirm the current findings and expand our understanding of what constitutes meaningful biomechanical change according to TTS scores in OA. The capability to stabilize one's posture after completing a dynamic movement is primarily based on how a person negotiates various physical constraints that result from neuroanatomical, biomechanical, and environmental origins. Thus, to better understand the neuromuscular system underlying postural control recovery strategies in OA, diverse factors, such as muscle power and psychiatric aspects (e.g., fear of falling), on postural control should be comprehensively considered in future studies.

Author Contributions: Conceptualization, H.L.; methodology, H.L.; writing—original draft preparation, H.L.; writing—review and editing, H.L. and K.B.; supervision, K.B.; project administration, H.L. and K.B. All authors have read and agreed to the published version of the manuscript.

Funding: This research received no external funding.

Institutional Review Board Statement: The study was conducted according to the guidelines of the Declaration of Helsinki, and approved by the Institutional Review Board of the University of Florida (IRB201401029).

Informed Consent Statement: Informed consent was obtained from all participants involved in the study.

Data Availability Statement: Not applicable.

Acknowledgments: We thank the study participants for their time and effort.

Conflicts of Interest: The authors declare no conflict of interest.

References

1. Murphy, S.L.; Williams, C.S.; Gill, T.M. Characteristics associated with fear of falling and activity restriction in community—Living older persons. *J. Am. Geriatr. Soc.* **2002**, *50*, 516–520. [CrossRef] [PubMed]
2. Maki, B.E.; McIlroy, W.E. Postural control in the older adult. *Clin. Geriatr. Med.* **1996**, *12*, 635–658. [CrossRef]
3. Oba, N.; Sasagawa, S.; Yamamoto, A.; Nakazawa, K. Difference in postural control during quiet standing between young children and adults: Assessment with center of mass acceleration. *PLoS ONE* **2015**, *10*, e0140235. [CrossRef]
4. Park, Y.S.; Kim, E.H.; Kim, T.W.; Lee, Y.S.; Lim, Y.T. The effects of 12-week balance ability improvement exercise to the changes of selected joint angles and ground reaction forces during down staircase walking. *Korean J. Sport Biomech.* **2010**, *20*, 267–275. [CrossRef]
5. Eun, S.D. An investigation of the effect of the height of wteps on the joint moment of lower extremities of the elderly while walking downstairs. *Korean J. Sport Biomech.* **2006**, *16*, 31–38.
6. Novak, A.C.; Brouwer, B. Kinematic and kinetic evaluation of the stance phase of stair ambulation in persons with stroke and healthy adults: A pilot study. *J. Appl. Biomech.* **2013**, *29*, 443–452. [CrossRef]
7. Startzell, J.K.; Owens, D.A.; Mulfinger, L.M.; Cavanagh, P.R. Stair negotiation in older people: A review. *J. Am. Geriatr Soc.* **2000**, *48*, 567–580. [CrossRef] [PubMed]
8. Granacher, U.; Muehlbauer, T.; Gruber, M. A qualitative review of balance and strength performance in healthy older adults: Impact for testing and training. *J. Aging Res.* **2012**, *2012*, 708905. [CrossRef] [PubMed]
9. Tinetti, M.E.; Speechley, M.; Ginter, S.F. Risk factors for falls among elderly persons living in the community. *N. Engl. J. Med.* **1988**, *319*, 1701–1707. [CrossRef]
10. Miyasike-daSilva, V.; McIlroy, W.E. Does it really matter where you look when walking on stairs? Insights from a dual-task study. *PLoS ONE* **2012**, *7*, e44722. [CrossRef]
11. Shin, S.; Jang, D.G.; Jang, J.K.; Park, S.H. The effect of age and dual task to human postural control. *Korean J. Sport Biomech.* **2013**, *23*, 169–177. [CrossRef]
12. Ojha, H.A.; Kern, R.W.; Lin, C.H.J.; Winstein, C.J. Age affects the attentional demands of stair ambulation: Evidence from a dual-task approach. *Phys. Ther.* **2009**, *89*, 1080–1088. [CrossRef] [PubMed]
13. Parihar, R.; Mahoney, J.R.; Verghese, J. Relationship of gait and cognition in the elderly. *Curr. Transl. Geriatr. Exp. Gerontol. Rep.* **2013**, *2*, 167–173. [CrossRef]
14. Ross, S.E.; Guskiewicz, K.M. Time to Stabilization: A Method for Analyzing Dynamic Postural Stability. *Int. J. Athl. Ther.* **2003**, *8*, 37–39.
15. Colby, S.; Hintermeister, R.A.; Torry, M.R.; Steadman, J.R. Lower limb stability with ACL impairment. *J. Orthop. Sports. Phys. Ther.* **1999**, *29*, 444–451. [CrossRef]
16. Prieto, T.E.; Myklebust, J.B.; Hoffmann, R.G.; Lovett, E.G.; Myklebust, B.M. Measures of postural steadiness: Differences between healthy young and elderly adults. *IEEE. Trans. Biomed. Eng.* **1996**, *43*, 956–966. [CrossRef] [PubMed]
17. Yamamoto, T.; Smith, C.E.; Suzuki, Y.; Kiyono, K.; Tanahashi, T.; Sakoda, S.; Morasso, P.; Nomura, T. Universal and individual characteristics of postural sway during quiet standing in healthy young adults. *Physiol. Rep.* **2015**, *3*, e12329.f. [CrossRef]
18. Vearrier, L.A.; Langan, J.; Shumway-Cook, A.; Woollacott, M. An intensive massed practice approach to retraining balance post-stroke. *Gait Posture* **2005**, *22*, 154–163. [CrossRef]
19. Bieryla, K.A.; Madigan, M.L. Proof of concept for perturbation-based balance training in older adults at a high risk for falls. *Arch. Phys. M. Arch. Phys. Med.* **2011**, *92*, 841–843. [CrossRef] [PubMed]
20. Lee, H.J.; Chou, L.S. Balance control during stair negotiation in older adults. *J. Biomech.* **2007**, *40*, 2530–2536. [CrossRef]
21. Reevesa, N.D.; Spanjaardab, M.; Mohagheghia, A.A.; Baltzopoulosa, V.; Maganarisa, C.N. Older adults employ alternative strategies to operate within their maximum capabilities when ascending stairs. *J. Electromyogr. Kinesiol.* **2009**, *19*, e57–e68. [CrossRef]

22. Shumway-Cook, A.; Baldwin, M.; Polisssar, N.L.; Gruber, W. Predicting the probability for falls in community-dwelling older adults. *Phys Ther.* **1997**, *77*, 812–819. [CrossRef]
23. Roman-Liu, D. Age-related changes in the range and velocity of postural sway. *Arch. Gerontol. Geriatr.* **2018**, *77*, 66–80. [CrossRef] [PubMed]
24. Lin, D.; Seol, H.; Nussbaum, M.A.; Madigan, M.L. Reliability of COP_based postural sway measures and age-related differences. *Gait Posture* **2008**, *28*, 337–342. [CrossRef] [PubMed]
25. Costigan, P.A.; Deluzio, K.J.; Wyss, U.P. Knee and hip kinetics during normal stair climbing. *Gait Posture* **2002**, *16*, 31–37. [CrossRef]
26. Della Croce, U.; Riley, P.O.; Lelas, J.L.; Kerrigan, D.C. A refined view of the determinants of gait. *Gait Posture* **2001**, *14*, 79–84. [CrossRef]
27. Shaw, M.Y.; Gribble, P.A.; Frye, J.L. Ankle bracing, fatigue, and time to stabilization in collegiate volleyball athletes. *J. Athl. Train.* **2008**, *43*, 164–171. [CrossRef] [PubMed]

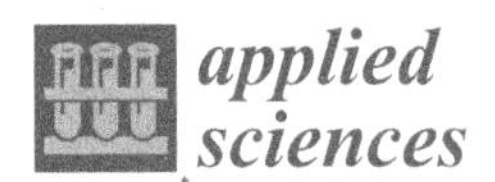

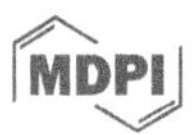

Article

Bilateral Deficits during Maximal Grip Force Production in Late Postmenopausal Women

Jin-Su Kim [1], Moon-Hyon Hwang [1,2] and Nyeonju Kang [1,3,4,*]

[1] Department of Human Movement Science, Graduate School, Incheon National University, Incheon 22012, Korea; jinsu.kim@ufl.edu (J.-S.K.); mhwang@inu.ac.kr (M.-H.H.)
[2] Division of Health & Kinesiology, Incheon National University, Incheon 22012, Korea
[3] Division of Sport Science, Sport Science Institute & Health Promotion Center, Incheon National University, Incheon 22012, Korea
[4] Neuromechanical Rehabilitation Research Laboratory, Incheon National University, Incheon 22012, Korea
* Correspondence: nyunju@inu.ac.kr; Tel.: +82-32-835-8573

Abstract: The purpose of this study was to investigate bilateral deficit patterns during maximal hand-grip force production in late postmenopausal women. Twenty late postmenopausal and 20 young premenopausal women performed maximal isometric grip force production tasks with dominant and nondominant hands and both hands, respectively. For late postmenopausal women, pulse wave analysis was used for identifying a potential relationship between maximal hand-grip strength and risk factors of cardiovascular disease. The findings showed that late postmenopausal women produced significantly decreased maximal hand-grip strength in dominant and nondominant and bilateral hand conditions compared to those of premenopausal women. Bilateral deficit patterns appeared in late postmenopausal women. For late postmenopausal women, decreased dominant and bilateral hand-grip forces were significantly related to greater bilateral deficit patterns. Further, less maximal hand-grip strength in unilateral and bilateral hand conditions correlated with greater central pulse pressure. These findings suggested that age-related impairments in muscle strength and estrogen deficiency may interfere with conducting successful activities of bilateral movements. Further, assessing maximal dominant hand-grip strength may predict bilateral deficit patterns and risk of cardiovascular disease in late postmenopausal women.

Keywords: bilateral deficit; postmenopausal; hand-grip strength; dominant hand; pulse wave analysis

Citation: Kim, J.-S.; Hwang, M.-H.; Kang, N. Bilateral Deficits during Maximal Grip Force Production in Late Postmenopausal Women. *Appl. Sci.* **2021**, *11*, 8426. https://doi.org/10.3390/app11188426

Academic Editor: Mark King

Received: 18 August 2021
Accepted: 8 September 2021
Published: 10 September 2021

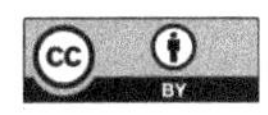

1. Introduction

Menopause typically occurs in women's 40s [1], and one third of women's lifespan is spent post-menopause [2]. Progressive reduction of estrogen in postmenopausal women may facilitate more age-related deficits in the central and peripheral nervous system [3–6]. For example, muscle weakness normally appears in elderly people because of age-induced neurophysiological alterations [7–9]. Furthermore, asymmetrical interlimb muscle strength interferes with executing bilateral movements that account for 54% of daily activities in the aging population [10,11]. Importantly, postmenopausal women reveal more significant reduction of muscle strength than premenopausal women and age-matched males [12–16].

Bilateral deficit is a phenomenon when individuals reveal lower force outputs produced simultaneously by both limbs than the sum of unilateral forces generated by each limb. Previous studies indicate that bilateral deficit may appear in either upper or lower extremities during various motor tasks such as maximal voluntary contraction (MVC), reaction time [17–19], and different contraction types (e.g., isometric and dynamic contraction) [20]. Moreover, greater levels of bilateral deficit are associated with increased impairment in bilateral performances (e.g., ballistic push-off and vertical squat jumping) [21–23], and several aging studies report bilateral deficit patterns in elderly people interfering with various functional movements (e.g., rising from a chair) [24,25].

For postmenopausal and elderly women, previous studies report bilateral deficit patterns in lower limb movements such as leg extension and leg press [24–28]. Specifically, greater bilateral deficit in producing explosive forces increases the time of sit-to-stand performance [25]. In postmenopausal women, increased interhemispheric inhibition and reduced muscle strength potentially induced by deficiency of estrogen and/or progesterone may facilitate bilateral deficit patterns [20,28,29]. However, these previous findings are mostly limited to lower limb movements. Given that successful bilateral upper limb movements are additional critical motor functions for older adults [11], determining whether bilateral deficit patterns in upper limb movements appear in late postmenopausal women is necessary. Thus, the purpose of this study was to examine bilateral deficit patterns in late postmenopausal women using voluntary maximal handgrip force tasks.

2. Materials and Methods

2.1. Particiapants

Twenty healthy late postmenopausal women (mean and standard deviation of age = 65.5 ± 3.1 years) and 20 healthy young premenopausal women (mean and standard deviation of age = 23.4 ± 2.1 years) participated in this study. We recruited participants using flyers in the university and local community centers and confirmed that all participants had no musculoskeletal deficits (e.g., sarcopenia) in their upper extremities, neurological disease, cardiovascular diseases, and significant cognitive impairments. Late postmenopausal women were defined as those with more than four years after menopause [30]. All participants were right-handed as assessed by the Edinburgh handedness inventory [31]. Specific details on demographic information are summarized in Table 1. Before starting the testing, all participants read and signed an informed consent form and experimental protocols approved by the University's Institutional Review Board.

Table 1. Demographic information.

Group	Late Postmenopausal Women	Young Premenopausal Women
Sample Size (n)	20	20
Age (years)	66 (63–73)	23 (22–25)
Handedness	20 right	20 right
Skeletal Muscle Mass (kg)	19.9 ± 1.6	23.6 ± 2.1
Body Fat Mass (kg)	20.6 ± 5.1	15.9 ± 4.0
Body Mass Index (kg/m^2)	23.9 ± 2.7	22.0 ± 2.3
Time Since Menopause (years)	14.4 ± 6.2	-
Central Pulse Pressure (mmHg)	35.6 ± 5.9	-
Augmentation index (%)	32.0 ± 7.5	-

Note. Data are mean ± standard deviation. Age data are median (interquartile range).

2.2. Experimental Setup

To investigate the bilateral deficit phenomenon in the upper extremities, we used an isometric hand-grip force production paradigm. Before executing isometric force production tasks, participants sat 80 cm away from a 54.6 cm LED monitor (1920 × 1080 pixels; refresh rate = 60 Hz, Dell, Round Rock, TX, USA) and maintained comfortable positions with 15–20° of shoulder flexion and 20–45° of elbow flexion. Using an isometric hand-grip force measurement system (SEED TECH Co., Ltd., Bucheon, Korea), participants grasped the handle (diameter = 30 mm) and produced their maximal isometric force outputs with their unilateral hand and both hands, respectively. Further, we instructed the participants to put their resting hand on the pad during the unilateral tasks and maintain their forearms fixed on the table with same position to avoid inadvertent force output caused by elbow, shoulder, or trunk movements.

We administered two consecutive maximal force production trials for each hand condition: (a) unilateral dominant hand (Figure 1a), (b) unilateral nondominant hand (Figure 1b), and (c) both hands (Figure 1c). For each trial, participants generated as much isometric hand-grip forces as possible for 3 s. They had 60 s of rest between trials and 180 s of rest between hand conditions. The mean of two maximal force production trials for each hand condition was used for further analysis.

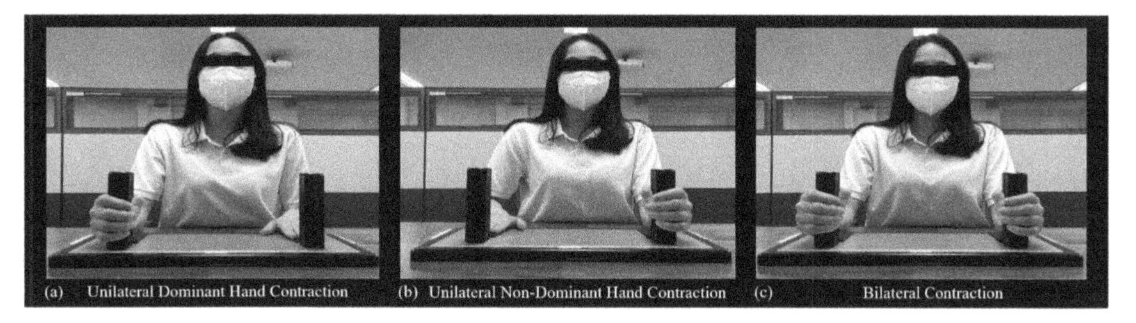

Figure 1. Hand-grip force production task. (**a**) Unilateral dominant hand contraction, (**b**) Unilateral nondominant hand contraction, and (**c**) Bilateral hands contraction.

Changes in handgrip strength in the aging population may be a risk factor indicating the occurrences of various cardiovascular diseases (e.g., hypertension, coronary artery disease, heart failure, or stroke) [32,33], and reduction of handgrip strength in elderly women is highly related to all-cause mortality [34]. Thus, for late postmenopausal women, we additionally performed non-invasive pulse wave analysis (PWA) using the SphygmoCor Xcel system (AtCor Medical, Sydney, Australia) to investigate the potential relationship between hand-grip force productions and cardiovascular disease risk factors. Before the PWA data collection, participants fasted for at least 10–12 h. All measurements proceeded in a light- and temperature-controlled room after resting for at least 10 min in the supine position. Participants wore a blood pressure cuff on their right upper arm to measure PWA. The blood pressure cuff automatically inflated to measure the brachial blood pressure and after deflating, it re-inflated to capture PWA waveforms. We conducted PWA at least three times, and the mean of two values which ranged within ±5 mmHg in blood pressure, ±5 beats/min in heart rate, and ±3% in augmentation index (AIx) was used for the further analysis.

2.3. Data Analysis

Bilateral index (%) of maximal handgrip force output (MF) was calculated by the following equations [35]. The values of bilateral index below zero indicate that bilateral motor performance was less than the sum of unilateral motor performance from each hand, so more negative values of bilateral index denote greater bilateral deficit patterns.

$$\text{Bilateral index } (\%) = \left(100 \times \frac{\text{Bilateral hands MF}}{(\text{Dominant hand MF} + \text{Non} - \text{dominant hand MF})}\right) - 100$$

Based on the brachial waveforms obtained from the blood pressure cuff, central aortic pressure waveforms were automatically calculated by the mathematical transfer function [36–38]. Central pulse pressure (cPP) is the difference between central systolic blood pressure (cSBP) and central diastolic blood pressure (cDBP). In addition, AIx (%), a measure of arterial stiffness, is calculated as the ratio of augmentation pressure (i.e., cSBP–inflection pressure) and cPP. Increased values of cPP and AIx may be related to a higher appearance rate of cardiovascular disease [39–41].

For statistical analyses, we performed an independent *t*-test to compare the differences of the bilateral index and maximal force production of unilateral hand and both hands between late postmenopausal and young premenopausal women. In addition, one sample *t*-test was used for determining whether the bilateral index for each group was significantly different from zero. For the late postmenopausal women group, Pearson's correlation analyses were performed to determine potential relations of maximal hand-grip forces of unilateral hand and both hands to bilateral deficit index as well as cardiovascular disease risk factors. Using the Shapiro–Wilk test, we confirmed that all dependent variables met the assumption of normality. Statistical analyses were performed using IBM SPSS Statistics version 25 (SPSS Inc, Chicago, IL, USA) with alpha set at 0.05.

3. Results

3.1. Maximal Hand-Grip Force Production

Maximal force production in late postmenopausal women was significantly lower than that in young premenopausal women, respectively, in the dominant hand ($t_{38} = -3.26$, $p = 0.002$), nondominant hand ($t_{38} = -2.26$, $p = 0.03$), and both hands ($t_{38} = -3.63$, $p = 0.001$; Figure 2A). Furthermore, the bilateral index values were significantly different between the late postmenopausal and young premenopausal women groups ($t_{38} = -2.68$, $p = 0.011$; Figure 2B). One sample t-test revealed that the bilateral index values in late postmenopausal women were significantly less than zero ($t_{19} = -2.24$, $p = 0.037$), indicating bilateral deficit patterns, whereas the bilateral index values in young premenopausal women were not significantly different from zero ($t_{19} = 1.59$, $p = 0.13$). These findings indicate that late postmenopausal women had reduced maximal hand-grip force in unilateral and bilateral tests and bilateral deficit patterns as compared to those in the young premenopausal women group.

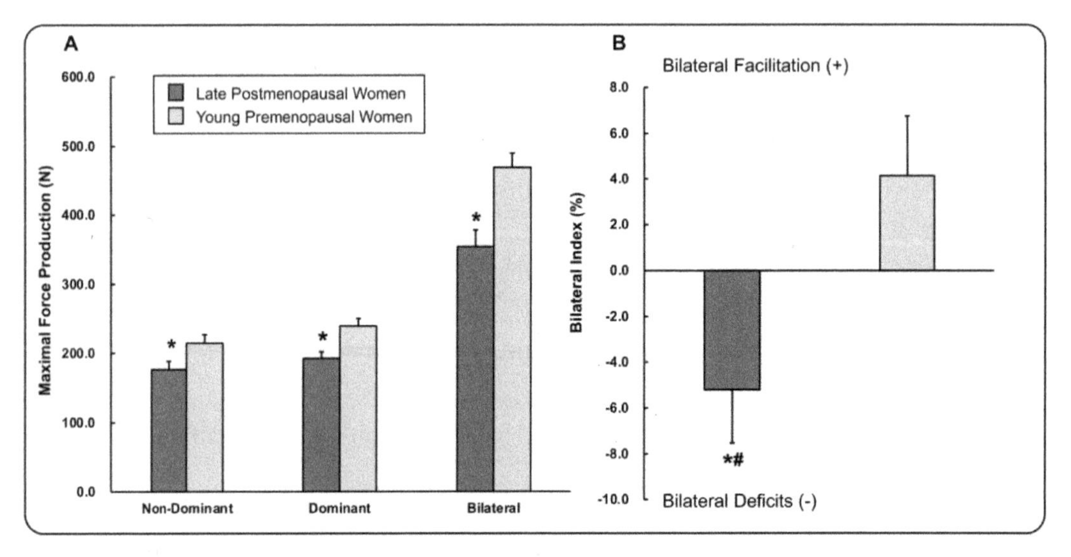

Figure 2. Maximal force production and bilateral index during isometric hand-grip force production tasks (M ± SE). (**A**) Maximal force production and (**B**) bilateral index. Asterisk (*) indicates significant difference ($p < 0.05$) between late postmenopausal and young premenopausal women. Number sign (#) indicates significant difference ($p < 0.05$) from zero.

3.2. Correlation Findings for Late Postmenopausal Women

Late postmenopausal women showed significant correlations between greater bilateral deficit patterns and more reduction of maximal hand-grip forces produced by the dominant hand and both hands, respectively (Table 2). Moreover, increased values of cPP were significantly related to less maximal hand-grip forces produced by the nondominant hand, dominant hand, and both hands, respectively. These findings indicate that decreased maximal hand-grip forces in the dominant hand and both hands were related to more bilateral deficit patterns and difference between cSBP and cDBP in late postmenopausal women.

Table 2. Correlation findings in late postmenopausal women.

	Bilateral Index	Central Pulse Pressure
Nondominant Hand MF	$r = 0.388; p = 0.091$	$r = -0.483; p = 0.031$ *
Dominant Hand MF	$r = 0.524; p = 0.018$ *	$r = -0.500; p = 0.025$ *
Bilateral Hand MF	$r = 0.705; p = 0.001$ *	$r = -0.510; p = 0.022$ *
Bilateral Index	-	$r = -0.280; p = 0.232$

Note: MF, maximal hand-grip force; asterisk (*) indicates $p < 0.05$.

4. Discussion

This study examined bilateral deficit patterns between late postmenopausal and young premenopausal women by estimating the maximal hand-grip force production. Late postmenopausal women showed significantly less hand-grip forces produced in both unilateral (i.e., dominant and nondominant hand) and bilateral tests, and further revealed greater bilateral deficit patterns than young premenopausal women. For late postmenopausal women, decreased maximal hand-grip forces generated by the dominant hand and both hands were significantly related to greater bilateral deficit patterns and increased values in central pulse pressure.

Despite inconsistent findings on the presence of a bilateral deficit pattern in the aging population [28,42], we found that a greater bilateral deficit in the upper extremities appeared in late postmenopausal women. These results expanded previous findings that mainly reported the bilateral deficit phenomenon in the lower extremities [24–28]. Reduced maximal hand-grip forces from each hand during bilateral contraction as compared to those during unilateral contraction may be related to higher interhemispheric inhibition between hemispheres in late menopausal women. Some previous studies asserted that bilateral deficit may be related to suppressive effects of interhemispheric inhibitions between hemispheres during bilateral movement execution [43,44]. In unimanual contraction, increased interhemispheric inhibition from the dominant hemisphere may influence the nondominant hemisphere to suppress the mirror movements of contralateral extremities [45,46]. In a bilateral contraction, both hemispheres may be affected by interhemispheric inhibitions, and these suppressions potentially interfere with motor outputs from each limb [47–49]. Interestingly, previous studies reported that greater levels of interhemispheric inhibition in premenopausal women were related to decreased estradiol level during the ovarian cycle, whereas these changes in interhemispheric inhibition level were not observed in males between pre- and post-tests with an interval of 14 days [50,51]. These findings raised a possibility that greater interhemispheric inhibition levels in late postmenopausal women induced by estrogen deficiency may be related to their bilateral deficit patterns during maximal hand-grip force production.

Moreover, our correlation findings indicated that greater reduction of maximal hand-grip strength in the dominant hand was significantly related to increased bilateral deficit patterns in late postmenopausal women. Previous studies reported that maximal hand-grip strength of the dominant hand in postmenopausal women significantly decreased as compared to those in either premenopausal women or age-matched men because of potential interactive effects of aging and estrogen deficiency [16,52]. Impaired muscle strength is frequently observed in older adults because of decreased muscle mass and quality (i.e., muscle strength per muscle mass) as referred to age-related sarcopenia [53]. Moreover, the occurrence rate of sarcopenia highly increases around 50s in women who may experience menopause [54,55]. Several studies posited that estrogen may show an anabolic effect on muscles by stimulating insulin-like growth factor-1 (IGF-1) receptors [56], and decreased levels of estrogen may be related to greater oxidative stress that potentially engenders muscle atrophy [57–59]. Moreover, postmenopausal women may have deficits in activation of estrogen receptors highly observed in type II muscle fibers [60,61] influenced by less estrogen and IGF-1 levels, and the deactivation of estrogen receptors presumably impairs muscle strength [58,62]. Consequently, estrogen deficiency in late postmenopausal women may facilitate functional impairments in the dominant hand related to increased bilateral deficits.

In addition, we found that higher cPP in late postmenopausal women was significantly related to less maximal hand-grip force produced by dominant and nondominant hand and both hands. Given the significant relationship between hand-grip force and muscle mass [63], our correlation findings support a proposition that sarcopenic older women showed higher levels of brachial pulse pressure than nonsarcopenic participants [64]. A potential mechanism underlying the relation of muscle mass to altered pulse pressure involves systemic inflammation markers. Increased circulating inflammation markers (e.g., c-reactive protein, interleukin–6, and tumor necrosis factor-alpha) were associated with reduced muscle strength and mass [65], and more inflammation markers may elevate pulse pressure by inducing endothelial dysfunction, increased arterial stiffness, and decreased nitric oxide bioavailability [66,67]. Higher pulse pressure is often associated with an increase of overall cardiovascular events and mortality of cardiovascular diseases [39,68]. Especially in postmenopausal women, managing risk factors of cardiovascular diseases is important because estrogen deficiency caused by menopause rapidly increases the risk of cardiovascular mortality [69]. Potentially, maximal hand-grip force production in either unilateral or bilateral conditions may additionally indicate risk of cardiovascular events in late postmenopausal women.

Although we found bilateral deficit patterns in late postmenopausal women, some limitations that should be cautiously interpreted remain in this study. First, we did not control the ovarian cycle and measure sex hormones in young premenopausal women. Given that estradiol concentrations are presumably related to levels of interhemispheric inhibition [50,51], different ovarian cycles in young premenopausal women might affect the bilateral index during maximal bilateral hand-grip contraction. Thus, future studies need to measure the bilateral index in young premenopausal women throughout the ovarian cycle to assess potential effect of estradiol levels on bilateral deficit patterns. Second, the current bilateral deficit patterns in late postmenopausal women may be influenced by interactive effects of aging and estrogen deficiency. To determine the potential effects of sex hormones on bilateral deficit patterns, future studies need to specify the relationship between altered levels of sex hormones and bilateral deficits in late postmenopausal women, and further test changes in bilateral deficits after hormone therapy interventions. Third, the lower levels of physical activity levels in late postmenopausal women may influence bilateral deficit patterns in their upper extremities, because older women with high levels of physical activity revealed greater muscle strength that potentially decreased bilateral deficit patterns [70]. Although we did not measure and specify different physical activity levels for late postmenopausal women, the potential relationship between physical activity and bilateral deficits in the upper extremities should be investigated in future studies. Lastly, in this study, we did not report the potential effects of greater bilateral deficits and less grip strength in the dominant hand on the execution of activities of daily living in late postmenopausal women. However, previous studies that focused on lower limb function found the relationship between greater bilateral deficits and more impaired daily living performances (e.g., rising from a chair) [24,25]. Despite no functional assessments on upper extremities for this study, further studies should determine whether bilateral deficit patterns in postmenopausal women are associated with activities of daily living requiring successful bimanual upper limb movements.

5. Conclusions

In conclusion, this study revealed bilateral deficit patterns in upper extremity for late postmenopausal women. Furthermore, decreased maximal hand-grip force production in the dominant hand was significantly related with greater bilateral deficit patterns for late postmenopausal women. Increased maximal hand-grip force in the dominant and non-dominant hands and both hands correlated with decreased central pulse pressure. These findings suggest that age-related impairments in muscle strength and estrogen deficiency in late postmenopausal women may interfere with conducting successful activities of bilateral movements. Moreover, estimating the dominant hand's maximal force production may provide beneficial information on progressive bilateral deficit patterns and risk factors of cardiovascular disease in late postmenopausal women.

Author Contributions: Conceptualization, M.-H.H. and N.K.; methodology, J.-S.K., M.-H.H. and N.K.; software, J.-S.K., M.-H.H. and N.K.; data curation, J.-S.K., M.-H.H. and N.K.; writing—original draft preparation, J.-S.K., M.-H.H. and N.K.; writing—review and editing, J.-S.K., M.-H.H. and N.K.; visualization, J.-S.K., M.-H.H. and N.K.; supervision, N.K.; project administration, N.K.; funding acquisition, N.K. All authors have read and agreed to the published version of the manuscript.

Funding: This research was funded by the National Research Foundation of Korea (NRF) grant funded by the Korea government (MSIT), grant number NRF-2018R1C1B5084455.

Institutional Review Board Statement: The study was conducted according to the guidelines of the Declaration of Helsinki and approved by the Institutional Review Board of Incheon National University (approval# 7007971-201810-002A and the study protocol was approved on 16 December 2020).

Informed Consent Statement: Informed consent was obtained from all subjects involved in the study.

Data Availability Statement: Not Available.

Acknowledgments: We thank the study participants for their time and effort.

Conflicts of Interest: The authors declare no conflict of interests.

References

1. Park, C.Y.; Lim, J.-Y.; Park, H.-Y. Age at natural menopause in Koreans: Secular trends and influences thereon. *Menopause* **2018**, *25*, 423–429. [CrossRef]
2. Global Aging into the 21st Century. 1996. Available online: https://www.census.gov/library/publications/1996/demo/96wchart.html (accessed on 18 August 2021).
3. Davy, K.P.; Desouza, C.A.; Jones, P.P.; Seals, D.R. Elevated heart rate variability in physically active young and older adult women. *Clin. Sci.* **1998**, *94*, 579–584. [CrossRef]
4. Huikuri, H.V.; Pikkujämsä, S.M.; Airaksinen, K.E.; Ikäheimo, M.J.; Rantala, A.O.; Kauma, H.; Lilja, M.; Kesäniemi, Y.A. Sex-related differences in autonomic modulation of heart rate in middle-aged subjects. *Circulation* **1996**, *94*, 122–125. [CrossRef] [PubMed]
5. Monteleone, P.; Mascagni, G.; Giannini, A.; Genazzani, A.R.; Simoncini, T. Symptoms of menopause—Global prevalence, physiology and implications. *Nat. Rev. Endocrinol.* **2018**, *14*, 199–215. [CrossRef]
6. Ribeiro, T.; Azevedo, G.; Crescêncio, J.; Marães, V.; Papa, V.; Catai, A.; Verzola, R.; Oliveira, L.; Silva de Sá, M.; Gallo, L., Jr. Heart rate variability under resting conditions in postmenopausal and young women. *Braz. J. Med. Biol. Res.* **2001**, *34*, 871–877. [CrossRef] [PubMed]
7. Ditroilo, M.; Forte, R.; Benelli, P.; Gambarara, D.; de Vito, G. Effects of age and limb dominance on upper and lower limb muscle function in healthy males and females aged 40–80 years. *J. Sports Sci.* **2010**, *28*, 667–677. [CrossRef] [PubMed]
8. Macaluso, A.; Nimmo, M.A.; Foster, J.E.; Cockburn, M.; McMillan, N.C.; de Vito, G. Contractile muscle volume and agonist-antagonist coactivation account for differences in torque between young and older women. *Muscle Nerve* **2002**, *25*, 858–863. [CrossRef]
9. Vandervoort, A.A. Aging of the human neuromuscular system. *Muscle Nerve* **2002**, *25*, 17–25. [CrossRef]
10. Beurskens, R.; Gollhofer, A.; Muehlbauer, T.; Cardinale, M.; Granacher, U. Effects of Heavy-Resistance Strength and Balance Training on Unilateral and Bilateral Leg Strength Performance in Old Adults. *PLoS ONE* **2015**, *10*, e0118535. [CrossRef]
11. Kilbreath, S.L.; Heard, R.C. Frequency of hand use in healthy older persons. *Aust. J. Physiother.* **2005**, *51*, 119–122. [CrossRef]
12. Calmels, P.; Vico, L.; Alexandre, C.; Minaire, P. Cross-sectional study of muscle strength and bone mineral density in a population of 106 women between the ages of 44 and 87 years: Relationship with age and menopause. *Eur. J. Appl. Physiol. Occup. Physiol.* **1995**, *70*, 180–186. [CrossRef] [PubMed]
13. Lindle, R.S.; Metter, E.J.; Lynch, N.A.; Fleg, J.L.; Fozard, J.L.; Tobin, J.; Roy, T.A.; Hurley, B.F. Age and gender comparisons of muscle strength in 654 women and men aged 20–93 yr. *J. Appl. Physiol.* **1997**, *83*, 1581–1587. [CrossRef]
14. Phillips, S.K.; Rook, K.M.; Siddle, N.C.; Bruce, S.A.; Woledge, R.C. Muscle weakness in women occurs at an earlier age than in men, but strength is preserved by hormone replacement therapy. *Clin. Sci.* **1993**, *84*, 95–98. [CrossRef]
15. Stanley, S.N.; Taylor, N.A.S. Isokinematic muscle mechanics in four groups of women of increasing age. *Eur. J. Appl. Physiol. Occup. Physiol.* **1993**, *66*, 178–184. [CrossRef]
16. Cipriani, C.; Romagnoli, E.; Carnevale, V.; Raso, I.; Scarpiello, A.; Angelozzi, M.; Tancredi, A.; Russo, S.; de Lucia, F.; Pepe, J.; et al. Muscle strength and bone in healthy women: Effect of age and gonadal status. *Hormones* **2012**, *11*, 325–332. [CrossRef] [PubMed]

17. Henry, F.M.; Smith, L.E. Simultaneous vs. Separate Bilateral Muscular Contractions in Relation to Neural Overflow Theory and Neuromoter Specificity. *Res. Q. Am. Assoc. Health Phys. Educ. Recreat.* **1961**, *32*, 42–46. [CrossRef]
18. Taniguchi, Y. Effect of practice in bilateral and unilateral reaction-time tasks. *Percept. Mot. Skills* **1999**, *88*, 99–109. [CrossRef]
19. Taniguchi, Y.; Burle, B.; Vidal, F.; Bonnet, M. Deficit in motor cortical activity for simultaneous bimanual responses. *Exp. Brain Res.* **2001**, *137*, 259–268. [CrossRef] [PubMed]
20. Škarabot, J.; Cronin, N.; Strojnik, V.; Avela, J. Bilateral deficit in maximal force production. *Eur. J. Appl. Physiol. Occup. Physiol.* **2016**, *116*, 2057–2084. [CrossRef] [PubMed]
21. Bobbert, M.F.; de Graaf, W.W.; Jonk, J.N.; Casius, L.J.R. Explanation of the bilateral deficit in human vertical squat jumping. *J. Appl. Physiol.* **2006**, *100*, 493–499. [CrossRef]
22. Samozino, P.; Rejc, E.; di Prampero, P.E.; Belli, A.; Morin, J.-B. Force–Velocity Properties' Contribution to Bilateral Deficit during Ballistic Push-off. *Med. Sci. Sports Exerc.* **2014**, *46*, 107–114. [CrossRef]
23. Van Dieen, J.H.; Ogita, F.; de Haan, A. Reduced Neural Drive in Bilateral Exertions: A Performance-Limiting Factor? *Med. Sci. Sports Exerc.* **2003**, *35*, 111–118. [CrossRef]
24. Pääsuke, M.; Ereline, J.; Gapeyeva, H.; Joost, K.; Mõttus, K.; Taba, P. Leg-Extension Strength and Chair-Rise Performance in Elderly Women with Parkinson's Disease. *J. Aging Phys. Act.* **2004**, *12*, 511–524. [CrossRef]
25. Ruiz-Cárdenas, J.; Rodríguez-Juan, J.; Jakobi, J.; Ríos-Díaz, J.; Marín-Cascales, E.; Rubio-Arias, J. Bilateral deficit in explosive force related to sit-to-stand performance in older postmenopausal women. *Arch. Gerontol. Geriatr.* **2018**, *74*, 145–149. [CrossRef]
26. Janzen, C.L.; Chilibeck, P.D.; Davison, K.S. The effect of unilateral and bilateral strength training on the bilateral deficit and lean tissue mass in post-menopausal women. *Eur. J. Appl. Physiol. Occup. Physiol.* **2006**, *97*, 253–260. [CrossRef] [PubMed]
27. Kuruganti, U.; Seaman, K. The bilateral leg strength deficit is present in old, young and adolescent females during isokinetic knee extension and flexion. *Eur. J. Appl. Physiol. Occup. Physiol.* **2006**, *97*, 322–326. [CrossRef] [PubMed]
28. Yamauchi, J.; Mishima, C.; Nakayama, S.; Ishii, N. Force–velocity, force–power relationships of bilateral and unilateral leg multi-joint movements in young and elderly women. *J. Biomech.* **2009**, *42*, 2151–2157. [CrossRef] [PubMed]
29. Bayer, U.; Hausmann, M. Estrogen treatment affects brain functioning after menopause. *Menopause Int.* **2011**, *17*, 148–152. [CrossRef]
30. Sherman, S. Defining the menopausal transition. *Am. J. Med.* **2005**, *118*, 3–7. [CrossRef] [PubMed]
31. Oldfield, R.C. The assessment and analysis of handedness: The Edinburgh inventory. *Neuropsychologia* **1971**, *9*, 97–113. [CrossRef]
32. Carbone, S.; Kirkman, D.L.; Garten, R.S.; Rodriguez-Miguelez, P.; Artero, E.G.; Lee, D.-C.; Lavie, C.J. Muscular strength and cardiovascular disease: An updated state-of-the-art narrative review. *J. Cardiopulm. Rehabil. Prev.* **2020**, *40*, 302–309. [CrossRef]
33. Leong, D.P.; Teo, K.K.; Rangarajan, S.; Lopez-Jaramillo, P.; Avezum, A., Jr.; Orlandini, A.; Seron, P.; Ahmed, S.H.; Rosengren, A.; Kelishadi, R. Prognostic value of grip strength: Findings from the Prospective Urban Rural Epidemiology (PURE) study. *Lancet* **2015**, *386*, 266–273. [CrossRef]
34. García-Hermoso, A.; Cavero-Redondo, I.; Ramírez Vélez, R.; Ruiz, J.R.; Ortega, F.B.; Lee, D.-C.; Martínez-Vizcaíno, V. Mus-cular strength as a predictor of all-cause mortality in an apparently healthy population: A systematic review and meta-analysis of data from approximately 2 million men and women. *Arch. Phys. Med. Rehabil.* **2018**, *99*, 2100–2113. [CrossRef] [PubMed]
35. Howard, J.D.; Enoka, R.M. Maximum bilateral contractions are modified by neurally mediated interlimb effects. *J. Appl. Physiol.* **1991**, *70*, 306–316. [CrossRef] [PubMed]
36. Butlin, M.; Qasem, A. Large artery stiffness assessment using SphygmoCor technology. *Pulse* **2016**, *4*, 180–192. [CrossRef]
37. Butlin, M.; Qasem, A.; Avolio, A.P. Estimation of central aortic pressure waveform features derived from the brachial cuff volume displacement waveform. In Proceedings of the 2012 Annual International Conference of the IEEE Engineering in Medicine and Biology Society, San Diego, CA, USA, 28 August–1 September 2012; pp. 2591–2594.
38. Karamanoglu, M.; O'Rourke, M.F.; Avolio, A.P.; Kelly, R.P. An analysis of the relationship between central aortic and peripheral upper limb pressure waves in man. *Eur. Heart J.* **1993**, *14*, 160–167. [CrossRef]
39. Roman, M.J.; Devereux, R.B.; Kizer, J.R.; Okin, P.M.; Lee, E.T.; Wang, W.; Umans, J.G.; Calhoun, D.; Howard, B.V. High Central Pulse Pressure Is Independently Associated with Adverse Cardiovascular Outcome: The Strong Heart Study. *J. Am. Coll. Cardiol.* **2009**, *54*, 1730–1734. [CrossRef] [PubMed]
40. Vlachopoulos, C.; Aznaouridis, K.; O'Rourke, M.F.; Safar, M.E.; Baou, K.; Stefanadis, C. Prediction of cardiovascular events and all-cause mortality with central haemodynamics: A systematic review and meta-analysis. *Eur. Heart J.* **2010**, *31*, 1865–1871. [CrossRef]
41. Weber, T.; Auer, J.; O'Rourke, M.F.; Kvas, E.; Laßnig, E.; Berent, R.; Eber, B. Arterial Stiffness, Wave Reflections, and the Risk of Coronary Artery Disease. *Circulation* **2004**, *109*, 184–189. [CrossRef] [PubMed]
42. Hernandez, J.P.; Nelson-Whalen, N.L.; Franke, W.D.; McLean, S.P. Bilateral index expressions and iEMG activity in older versus young adults. *J. Gerontol. Ser. A Boil. Sci. Med. Sci.* **2003**, *58*, M536–M541. [CrossRef]
43. Perez, M.A.; Butler, J.E.; Taylor, J.L. Modulation of transcallosal inhibition by bilateral activation of agonist and antagonist proximal arm muscles. *J. Neurophysiol.* **2014**, *111*, 405–414. [CrossRef]
44. Soteropoulos, D.S.; Perez, M.A. Physiological changes underlying bilateral isometric arm voluntary contractions in healthy humans. *J. Neurophysiol.* **2011**, *105*, 1594–1602. [CrossRef]
45. Cincotta, M.; Ziemann, U. Neurophysiology of unimanual motor control and mirror movements. *Clin. Neurophysiol.* **2008**, *119*, 744–762. [CrossRef]

46. Vercauteren, K.; Pleysier, T.; van Belle, L.; Swinnen, S.P.; Wenderoth, N. Unimanual muscle activation increases interhe-mispheric inhibition from the active to the resting hemisphere. *Neurosci. Lett.* **2008**, *445*, 209–213. [CrossRef]
47. DeJong, S.L.; Lang, C.E. The bilateral movement condition facilitates maximal but not submaximal paretic-limb grip force in people with post-stroke hemiparesis. *Clin. Neurophysiol.* **2012**, *123*, 1616–1623. [CrossRef] [PubMed]
48. Oda, S.; Moritani, T. Movement-related cortical potentials during handgrip contractions with special reference to force and electromyogram bilateral deficit. *Eur. J. Appl. Physiol. Occup. Physiol.* **1995**, *72*, 1–5. [CrossRef] [PubMed]
49. Oda, S.; Moritani, T. Cross-correlation studies of movement-related cortical potentials during unilateral and bilateral muscle contractions in humans. *Eur. J. Appl. Physiol. Occup. Physiol.* **1996**, *74*, 29–35. [CrossRef]
50. Weis, S.; Hausmann, M. Sex Hormones: Modulators of Interhemispheric Inhibition in the Human Brain. *Neuroscience* **2009**, *16*, 132–138. [CrossRef] [PubMed]
51. Weis, S.; Hausmann, M.; Stoffers, B.; Vohn, R.; Kellermann, T.; Sturm, W. Estradiol Modulates Functional Brain Organization during the Menstrual Cycle: An Analysis of Interhemispheric Inhibition. *J. Neurosci.* **2008**, *28*, 13401–13410. [CrossRef]
52. Lee, J.E.; Kim, K.W.; Paik, N.-J.; Jang, H.C.; Chang, C.B.; Baek, G.H.; Lee, Y.H.; Gong, H.S. Evaluation of Factors Influencing Grip Strength in Elderly Koreans. *J. Bone Metab.* **2012**, *19*, 103–110. [CrossRef] [PubMed]
53. Cruz-Jentoft, A.J.; Baeyens, J.P.; Bauer, J.M.; Boirie, Y.; Cederholm, T.; Landi, F.; Martin, F.C.; Michel, J.-P.; Rolland, Y.; Schneider, S.M.; et al. Sarcopenia: European consensus on definition and diagnosis: Report of the European Working Group on Sarcopenia in Older People. *Age Ageing* **2010**, *39*, 412–423. [CrossRef]
54. Aloia, J.F.; McGowan, D.M.; Vaswani, A.N.; Ross, P.; Cohn, S.H. Relationship of menopause to skeletal and muscle mass. *Am. J. Clin. Nutr.* **1991**, *53*, 1378–1383. [CrossRef] [PubMed]
55. Janssen, I.; Heymsfield, S.B.; Ross, R. Low relative skeletal muscle mass (sarcopenia) in older persons is associated with func-tional impairment and physical disability. *J. Am. Geriatr. Soc.* **2002**, *50*, 889–896. [CrossRef] [PubMed]
56. Sitnick, M.; Foley, A.M.; Brown, M.; Spangenburg, E.E. Ovariectomy prevents the recovery of atrophied gastrocnemius skeletal muscle mass. *J. Appl. Physiol.* **2006**, *100*, 286–293. [CrossRef] [PubMed]
57. Jackson, M.J. Interactions Between Reactive Oxygen Species Generated by Contractile Activity and Aging in Skeletal Muscle? *Antioxid. Redox Signal.* **2013**, *19*, 804–812. [CrossRef]
58. Maltais, M.L.; Desroches, J.; Dionne, I.J. Changes in muscle mass and strength after menopause. *J. Musculoskelet. Neuronal Interact.* **2009**, *9*, 186–197.
59. Powers, S.K.; Jackson, M.J. Exercise-Induced Oxidative Stress: Cellular Mechanisms and Impact on Muscle Force Production. *Physiol. Rev.* **2008**, *88*, 1243–1276. [CrossRef]
60. Brown, M. Skeletal muscle and bone: Effect of sex steroids and aging. *Adv. Physiol. Educ.* **2008**, *32*, 120–126. [CrossRef]
61. Wiik, A.; Ekman, M.; Johansson, O.; Jansson, E.; Esbjörnsson, M. Expression of both oestrogen receptor alpha and beta in human skeletal muscle tissue. *Histochem. Cell Biol.* **2008**, *131*, 181–189. [CrossRef]
62. Pfeilschifter, J.; Scheidt-Nave, C.; Leidig-Bruckner, G.; Woitge, H.W.; Blum, W.F.; Wüster, C.; Haack, D.; Ziegler, R. Relationship between circulating insulin-like growth factor components and sex hormones in a population-based sample of 50-to 80-year-old men and women. *J. Clin. Endocrinol. Metab.* **1996**, *81*, 2534–2540.
63. Kallman, D.A.; Plato, C.C.; Tobin, J.D. The Role of Muscle Loss in the Age-Related Decline of Grip Strength: Cross-Sectional and Longitudinal Perspectives. *J. Gerontol.* **1990**, *45*, M82–M88. [CrossRef]
64. Coelho, H.J., Jr.; Aguiar, S.; Gonçalves, I.D.O.; Sampaio, R.A.C.; Uchida, M.C.; Moraes, M.R.; Asano, R.Y. Sarcopenia Is Associated with High Pulse Pressure in Older Women. *J. Aging Res.* **2015**, *2015*, 1–6. [CrossRef] [PubMed]
65. Tuttle, C.S.; Thang, L.A.; Maier, A.B. Markers of inflammation and their association with muscle strength and mass: A sys-tematic review and meta-analysis. *Ageing Res. Rev.* **2020**, *64*, 101185. [CrossRef] [PubMed]
66. Jain, S.; Khera, R.; Corrales-Medina, V.F.; Townsend, R.R.; Chirinos, J.A. "Inflammation and arterial stiffness in humans". *Atherosclerosis* **2014**, *237*, 381–390. [CrossRef]
67. Zhang, C. The role of inflammatory cytokines in endothelial dysfunction. *Basic Res. Cardiol.* **2008**, *103*, 398–406. [CrossRef] [PubMed]
68. Said, M.A.; Eppinga, R.N.; Lipsic, E.; Verweij, N.; van der Harst, P. Relationship of Arterial Stiffness Index and Pulse Pressure with Cardiovascular Disease and Mortality. *J. Am. Heart Assoc.* **2018**, *7*, e007621. [CrossRef]
69. Lewis, S.J. Cardiovascular disease in postmenopausal women: Myths and reality. *Am. J. Cardiol.* **2002**, *89*, 5–10. [CrossRef]
70. Martin, H.J.; Syddall, H.E.; Dennison, E.M.; Cooper, C.; Sayer, A.A. Relationship between customary physical activity, muscle strength and physical performance in older men and women: Findings from the Hertfordshire Cohort Study. *Age Ageing* **2008**, *37*, 589–593. [CrossRef]

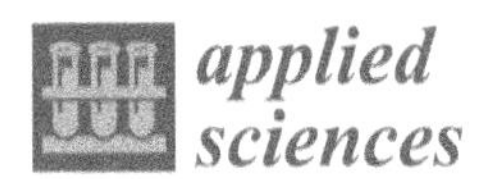
applied sciences

MDPI

Article

Effect of Limb-Specific Resistance Training on Central and Peripheral Artery Stiffness in Young Adults: A Pilot Study

Minyoung Kim [1], Ruda Lee [1], Nyeonju Kang [2,3] and Moon-Hyon Hwang [3,4,*]

[1] Department of Human Movement Science, Graduate School, Incheon National University, Incheon 22012, Korea; sks911222@naver.com (M.K.); winner72@inu.ac.kr (R.L.)
[2] Division of Sport Science, Incheon National University, Incheon 22012, Korea; nyunju@inu.ac.kr
[3] Sport Science Institute, Incheon National University, Incheon 22012, Korea
[4] Division of Health & Kinesiology, Incheon National University, Incheon 22012, Korea
* Correspondence: mhwang@inu.ac.kr; Tel.: +82-32-835-8698

Abstract: This study aimed to investigate the effect of limb-specific resistance training on arterial stiffness in young adults. Twenty-four participants were randomly assigned to three groups: upper-limb resistance training (n = 8 (URT)), lower-limb resistance training (n = 8 (LRT)), and control group (n = 8 (CON)). Both URT and LRT groups performed the limb-specific resistance training at 70–80% of one-repetition maximum twice a week for 8 weeks. The aortic pulse wave velocity and augmentation index (AIx) were measured by the SphygmoCor XCEL to assess central artery stiffness. Peripheral artery stiffness was evaluated by brachial to radial artery pulse wave velocity (ArmPWV) and femoral to posterior tibial artery pulse wave velocity (LegPWV) using Doppler flowmeters. URT significantly reduced AIx (4.7 ± 3.0 vs. 0.3 ± 2.9%, pre vs. post, P = 0.01), and ArmPWV presented a tendency to decrease following URT (10.4 ± 0.3 vs. 8.6 ± 0.8 m/s, pre vs. post, P = 0.06). LRT showed no negative influence on central and peripheral artery stiffness. Changes in serum triglyceride and leg lean body mass after resistance training were significantly associated with changes in AIx and LegPWV, respectively. URT is beneficial in decreasing central artery wave reflection and may help to improve local peripheral artery stiffness even in healthy young adults.

Keywords: resistance training; arterial stiffness; pulse wave velocity; augmentation index

Citation: Kim, M.; Lee, R.; Kang, N.; Hwang, M.-H. Effect of Limb-Specific Resistance Training on Central and Peripheral Artery Stiffness in Young Adults: A Pilot Study. *Appl. Sci.* **2021**, *11*, 2737. https://doi.org/10.3390/app11062737

Academic Editors: Monica Gallo and Antonio Scarano

Received: 5 January 2021
Accepted: 12 March 2021
Published: 18 March 2021

1. Introduction

Cardiovascular disease (CVD) is the leading cause of death, and arterial stiffness is an early marker of CVD risk [1]. Large elastic arteries buffer augmented pulsatile energy and blood pressure when the heart pumps blood into the systemic vascular network [2]. Thus, an increase in large elastic artery stiffness augments central blood pressure and left ventricular load, which in turn reduces coronary artery perfusion and may increase acute cardiac event risk [3,4]. Even in young adults, a decrease in arterial distensibility, a measure of arterial stiffness, increases the number of cardiovascular risk factors [5].

Both aerobic and resistance exercises are recommended to prevent chronic diseases and to promote overall health in various populations [6–12]. Regular aerobic exercise is a well-known intervention to reduce blood pressure and arterial stiffness [13–15]. Resistance exercise is a typical physical activity and is commonly prescribed to enhance musculoskeletal and cardiovascular function [16,17]. Compared to its superior effect on musculoskeletal function and metabolic efficiency, the effect of resistance training on cardiovascular function, particularly arterial stiffness, is still controversial. Miyachi et al. reported that long-term resistance training decreased arterial stiffness in young and middle-aged men [18], but another previous finding demonstrated that resistance training impaired arterial stiffness, including carotid artery compliance [19]. Regarding training intensity, low-intensity resistance exercise decreased arterial stiffness, whereas moderate- to high-intensity resistance exercise augmented arterial stiffness in healthy young adults [20–24].

Furthermore, previous studies have hardly investigated thoroughly the benefit of limb-specific resistance exercise on both central and peripheral artery stiffness with validated vascular size-specific (central vs. peripheral) research methods. Thus, the purpose of this study was to examine the effect of limb-specific resistance training on both central and peripheral artery stiffness in healthy young adults.

2. Materials and Methods

2.1. Participants

Twenty-five young adults volunteered to participate in this study. They had not been doing any regular resistance training (that is, any type of resistance exercise for more than 2 days a week) for at least 6 months. Participants were excluded from this study if they had a smoking history in the last 5 years; any overt clinical diseases, including CVD, diabetes, and metabolic syndrome; or musculoskeletal problems that limit resistance exercises. A total of 24 participants (9 men and 15 women; 18–25 years old) finished this study, except for 1 participant who sustained a muscular injury unrelated to this study. Each participant voluntarily signed an informed consent after a thorough explanation of the nature, purposes, and risks of the study. The Institutional Review Board of Incheon National University approved this study. The study was conducted in accordance with the ethical standards of the Declaration of Helsinki.

2.2. Study Design

The study participants were randomly assigned to three groups: nonexercise control ((CON) $n = 8$), upper-limb resistance training ((URT) $n = 8$), and lower-limb resistance training ((LRT) $n = 8$). The participants in the CON group were asked to maintain their normal lifestyle for 8 weeks. The young adults in the URT and LRT groups were required to maintain their normal lifestyle and to complete the scheduled resistance exercise sessions. At both pre- and post-training, physiological parameters were obtained in a supine position in a temperature-controlled and semidarkened room and taken at the same time in the morning after at least 10 h of an overnight fast. To minimize the acute effect of resistance exercise, post-training measures were performed 20 to 24 h after finishing the last exercise session in the training groups. All physiological measures on female participants were performed in the early follicular phase to exclude the confounding effects of sex hormones on vascular function. All research procedures and supervised resistance exercise sessions were implemented in the Exercise & Cardiovascular Physiology Laboratory at Incheon National University.

2.3. Height, Weight, and Body Composition

The participants' height was measured in mm using a stadiometer. Body weight, fat mass, percent body fat, body mass index, and lean body mass (LBM) were evaluated by a segmental bioelectrical impedance analysis device (Inbody 720, Biospace, Seoul, Korea).

2.4. Central Artery Stiffness

Augmentation index (AIx) and aortic pulse wave velocity (AorPWV), which are validated, noninvasive measures of arterial stiffness, were evaluated by the SphygmoCor XCEL system (AtCor Medical, Sydney, Australia) [25–28]. The participants rested in a supine position for 15 min prior to the measurements following at least 10 h of overnight fast. To measure AIx, brachial artery pressure waveforms were obtained by a blood pressure cuff placed on the right upper arm. The brachial waveforms were then automatically transformed into central artery waveforms by the mathematical transfer function embedded in the system. The system estimated AIx as the ratio of amplified systolic blood pressure to pulse pressure in the central artery. AorPWV, which is a reliable, noninvasive measure of arterial stiffness in humans, was assessed by simultaneously measuring the carotid pulse waveforms by applanation tonometry and the femoral pulse waveforms by a blood pressure cuff placed on the right upper leg proximal to the inguinal ligament [28,29]. In the system, AorPWV was automatically calculated as the ratio of the distance between the two arterial measuring sites and the time of pulse waves moving between these two sites. The average of the three high-quality measures was used for AIx and AorPWV. The distance between the carotid and femoral artery measuring site was defined as previously mentioned [28]. In our laboratory, the day-to-day intertest coefficients of variation for AorPWV and AIx measurements were 4.4% and 11.2%, respectively.

2.5. Peripheral Artery Stiffness

A transcutaneous Doppler flowmeter (model 810-A, Parks Medical Electronics, Inc., Aloha, OR, USA) was employed to measure arm pulse wave velocity (ArmPWV) and leg pulse wave velocity (LegPWV). Pressure waves measured at the peripheral artery sites were digitized with a signal processing data acquisition system (model PL2604, AD Instruments Inc., Colorado Springs, CO, USA). Through an offline analysis, PWV was calculated as the distance in meters divided by the pulse transit time in seconds between the two recording sites. ArmPWV and LegPWV were determined by taking the average of the PWVs obtained from 10 paired pressure waveforms in the brachial and radial arteries and in the femoral and posterior tibial arteries, respectively. Due to the technical difficulty in measuring the high-quality arterial pressure waveforms at the two recording sites at the same time, electrocardiogram R-waves simultaneously measured with the pressure waveforms were used as a reference mark when calculating the pulse transit time between the two recording sites.

2.6. Blood Chemistry

To analyze the effects of resistance training on traditional CVD risk, serum triglyceride was analyzed by the enzymatic colorimetric assay using a triglycerides assay kit (TRIGL, Roche, Germany) and the Cobas 8000 analyzer (c702, Roche, Germany) pre- and post-training. The blood concentrations of epinephrine and norepinephrine were assessed by high-performance liquid chromatography (Acclaim, Bio-Rad, Hercules, CA, USA) using a plasma catecholamines assay kit (Plasma Catecholamines by HPLC, Bio-Rad, Feldkirchen, Germany) to investigate changes in the autonomic nervous system function and related hormones after the scheduled resistance exercise sessions. All of the blood chemistries were performed within a clinical laboratory. To avoid the influence of invasive blood from drawing on other physiological measures, the blood collection was performed following other physiological measures pre- and post-training.

2.7. Maximal Strength

The maximal strength of one-repetition maximum (1 RM) for chest and shoulder press, seated row, and barbell curl exercise was measured during URT, and 1 RM for leg extension, leg press, lying leg curl, and hip extension exercise was evaluated for LRT. In this study, 1 RM for each exercise was determined by an indirect estimation equation after pre- and post-training measures to maximize safety as previously described [30]. To summarize, the participants performed warm-up and stretching exercises for 5 min prior to the test. The warm-up exercise was composed of resistance exercises with a load of about 10 RM. In the test, the weight load was progressively increased to 2–5 RM load with a 3-min rest after beginning the test with 8–10 RM load. The indirect estimation equation for 1 RM was presented as W0 + W1. In this equation, W0 indicates the weight load considered to be slightly heavy by the participants between 2 and 8 RM load, and W1 means the following calculation: W0 × 0.025 × the number of repetitions.

2.8. Resistance Training Program

URT and LRT groups performed the scheduled resistance exercise sessions 2 days a week (either Monday and Wednesday or Tuesday and Thursday) for 8 weeks using an air resistance weight machine system (HUR Oy, Kokkola, Finland). The resistance training program was established to perform 4 exercises per session, 5 sets per exercise, and

10 repetitions per set with 2 min of rest between sets and exercises. The resistance training program for URT consisted of chest and shoulder press, seated row, and barbell curl exercises. Leg extension, lying curl, leg press, and hip extension exercises were included in the LRT program. Exercise intensity was set between 70 and 80% of 1 RM in each resistance exercise; the intensity between the 1st and 4th week was established at 70% of 1 RM and was adjusted to 80% of 1 RM thereafter. All of the exercise sessions were supervised by an exercise physiologist who provided verbal motivation and feedback.

2.9. Statistical Analyses

Statistical analyses were performed using an SPSS Statistics program (version 24, IBM SPSS Inc., Armonk, NY, USA). A one-way analysis of variance was used to examine whether pre-intervention group differences existed or not. In each group, the effect of intervention on the main dependent variables was evaluated by a paired t-test. Relationships between changes in arterial stiffness and other physiological variables were assessed using Pearson's correlation coefficient because all data included in this correlation analysis were normally distributed. Statistical significance was set at $P < 0.05$.

3. Results

The participants' characteristics are presented in Table 1.

Table 1. Participant characteristics pre- and post-intervention.

Variables	CON (n = 8)		URT (n = 8)		LRT (n = 8)	
	Pre	Post	Pre	Post	Pre	Post
Age, years	21 ± 1	-	20 ± 1	-	20 ± 1	-
Height, cm	164.4 ± 1.2	-	172.8 ± 4.7	-	170.2 ± 2.0	-
Weight, kg	60.0 ± 3.3	59.0 ± 3.5	65.0 ± 4.9	67.6 ± 5.7	65.1 ± 3.6	63.4 ± 4.0
BMI, kg/m^2	21.8 ± 1.1	21.8 ± 1.2	21.5 ± 0.6	21.9 ± 0.7	22.4 ± 0.9	22.7 ± 1.0
Body fat, %	23.1 ± 2.5	23.9 ± 2.3	18.5 ± 2.4	17.4 ± 2.5	24.3 ± 2.2	25.8 ± 2.4
Muscle mass, kg	25.0 ± 1.3	24.8 ± 1.2	30.2 ± 3.4	31.0 ± 3.4 *	27.6 ± 2.2	28.1 ± 2.1
Trunk LBM, kg	20.0 ± 1.0	19.7 ± 0.9	22.4 ± 2.0	23.2 ± 2.2 *	20.9 ± 1.4	21.3 ± 1.4 *
Arm LBM, kg	2.3 ± 0.2	2.2 ± 0.2	2.6 ± 0.3	2.8 ± 0.4 *	2.4 ± 0.2	2.4 ± 0.2 *
Leg LBM, kg	7.0 ± 0.3	7.1 ± 0.3	8.7 ± 1.1	8.8 ± 1.0	8.0 ± 0.6	8.1 ± 0.6
rHR, beat/min	59 ± 3	58 ± 2	58 ± 3	52 ± 2 *	57 ± 3	53 ± 3
SBP, mmHg	110 ± 2	111 ± 4	115 ± 4	114 ± 4	113 ± 3	109 ± 4
DBP, mmHg	64 ± 2	64 ± 2	64 ± 2	61 ± 3	63 ± 1	63 ± 3
Triglyc, mg/dL	64 ± 6	74 ± 13	66 ± 8	67 ± 7	71 ± 11	72 ± 12
Epi, pg/mL	43 ± 2	35 ± 3	41 ± 2	32 ± 3	52 ± 7	34 ± 3
Norepi, pg/mL	325 ± 33	128 ± 14 *	413 ± 36	140 ± 15 *	372 ± 25	118 ± 19 *

Data are mean ± SE. Abbreviations: CON, nontraining control group; URT, upper-limb resistance training group; LRT, lower-limb resistance training group; BMI, body mass index; LBM, lean body mass; rHR, resting heart rate; SBP, systolic blood pressure; DBP, diastolic blood pressure; Triglyc, triglycerides; Epi, epinephrine; Norepi, norepinephrine. There was no significant group difference at pre-intervention. * $P \leq 0.05$ vs. pre-intervention.

No significant difference was noted in age, weight, heart rate and blood pressure, and blood lipid and catecholamine levels among the CON, URT, and LRT groups prior to the intervention ($P \geq 0.16$; Table 1). No significant difference was observed in body composition parameters, including weight, body mass index, percent body fat, muscle mass, and segmental (trunk, arm, and leg) LBM, among the three groups at baseline ($P \geq 0.21$; Table 1). As expected, the abovementioned body composition factors did not change in the CON group after maintaining a nonexercise lifestyle during the intervention. The URT group had a significant improvement in muscle mass and arm LBM ($P \leq 0.01$); however, the LRT group showed no improvement in muscle mass and leg LBM after the established intervention ($P \geq 0.12$; Table 1). An increased trunk LBM was observed in the URT and LRT groups following the training ($P \leq 0.02$; Table 1). As a result of resistance training, the maximal strength of every exercise in both URT and LRT groups significantly improved between 14.0 and 24.3% ($P \leq 0.006$; Table 2).

Table 2. Changes in maximal strength (1 RM) after resistance training.

Group	Exercise	Pre-Intervention	Post-Intervention	*t*-Test *P* Value	Δ1 RM (%)
URT	Chest press, kg	66.8 ± 3.0	81.7 ± 2.9	0.0001	22.3
	Shoulder press, kg	58.5 ± 8.4	71.2 ± 11.1	0.006	21.7
	Seated row, kg	20.2 ± 1.2	23.3 ± 0.5	0.004	15.3
	Barbell curl, kg	24.3 ± 2.8	30.2 ± 2.7	0.0001	24.3
LRT	Leg press, kg	182.7 ± 14.0	208.3 ± 14.8	0.001	14.0
	Leg extension, kg	78.4 ± 5.6	93.8 ± 4.3	0.0001	19.6
	Lying leg curl, kg	15.4 ± 1.7	18.8 ± 1.7	0.0001	22.1
	Hip extension, kg	13.9 ± 1.7	16.4 ± 1.7	0.0001	18.0

Data are mean ± SE. Abbreviations: RM, repetition maximum; URT, upper-limb resistance training group; LRT, lower-limb resistance training group.

In response to the 8-week intervention, AIx was significantly reduced in the URT group ($P = 0.01$; Figure 1A), but no change was noted in the LRT and CON groups. URT and LRT did not lead to a significant change in AorPWV compared to the baseline value (Figure 1B). ArmPWV showed a tendency to decrease following URT, but this tendency did not reach statistical significance ($P = 0.06$; Figure 1C). No change was observed in the LegPWV following LRT (Figure 1D).

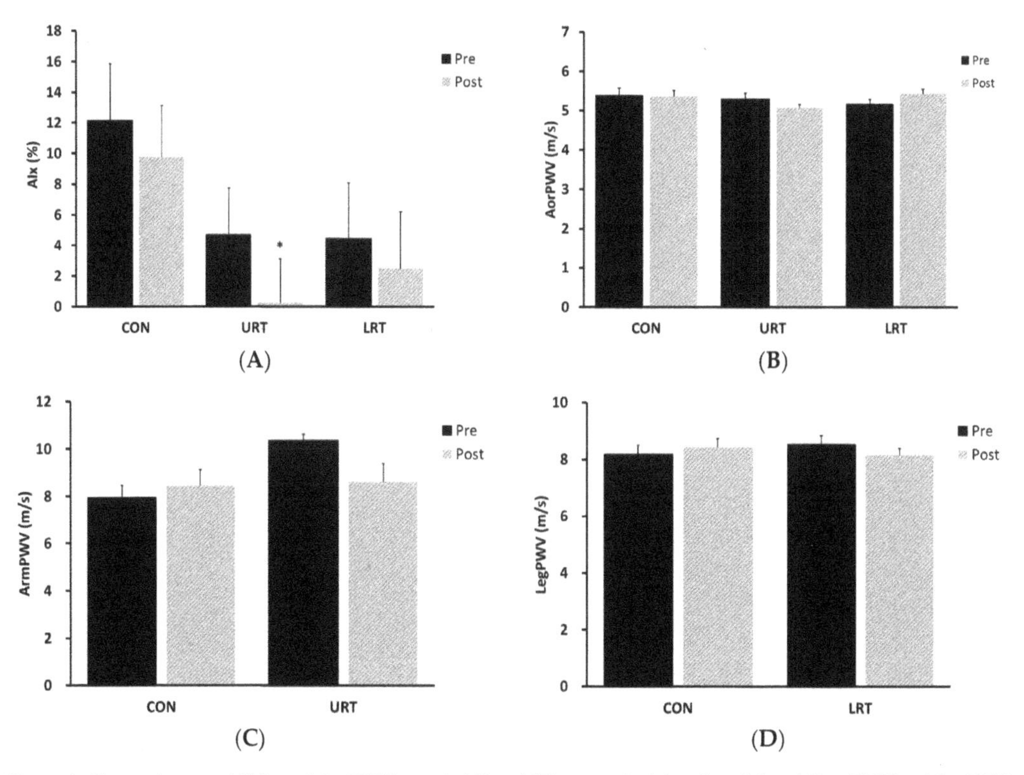

Figure 1. Change in central (AIx and AorPWV, panels (**A**) and (**B**), respectively) and peripheral (ArmPWV and LegPWV, panels (**C**) and (**D**), respectively) artery stiffness in response to the intervention. AIx, augmentation index; AorPWV, aortic (carotid–femoral artery) pulse wave velocity; ArmPWV, arm (brachial–radial artery) pulse wave velocity, LegPWV, leg (femoral–posterior tibial artery) pulse wave velocity; CON, nontraining control group; URT, upper-limb resistance training group; LRT, lower-limb resistance training group.

Plasma epinephrine concentration tended to decrease in the three groups but showed no statistical significance ($P \geq 0.07$; Table 1). The norepinephrine level was significantly reduced in all groups ($P \leq 0.001$; Table 1). In the resistance training groups, changes in AIx and LegPWV were significantly associated with changes in serum triglyceride levels and leg LBM, respectively (r = 0.57 and −0.61, P = 0.02 and 0.01; Figure 2). The changes in AorPWV and trunk LBM in response to resistance training seemed related to each other but did not reach statistical significance (r = 0.41, P = 0.06).

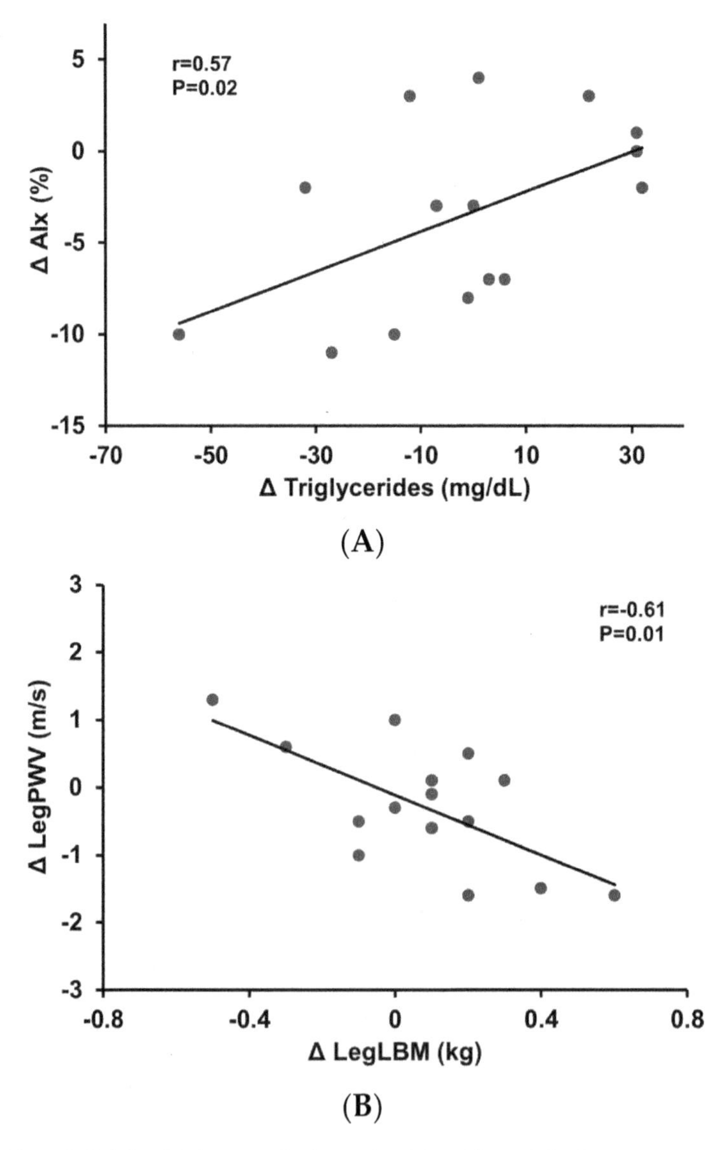

Figure 2. Relationship between the change in triglycerides and the change in augmentation index in response to resistance training (panel (**A**)). Relationship between the change in leg lean body mass and the change in leg pulse wave velocity in response to resistance training (panel (**B**)). AIx, augmentation index; PWV, pulse wave velocity; LBM, lean body mass.

4. Discussion

This study was performed to investigate the effect of limb-specific resistance training on both central and peripheral artery stiffness in young adults. It is, to our knowledge, the first to assess the effect of limb-specific long-term resistance training on both central and peripheral artery stiffness in young adults without any clinical disease.

Resistance exercise is one type of exercise recommended for improving muscular strength and cardiovascular function and for preventing musculoskeletal diseases, such as osteopenia and osteoporosis [31]. Although resistance exercise is recommended to enhance cardiovascular health, the effect of resistance exercise on arterial stiffness is still controversial. In this study, 8 weeks of URT reduced AIx, but not AorPWV, in young adults. For the same duration, LRT did not change the central artery stiffness measures. It has been documented that change in the resting heart rate after exercise training influences AIx, which may result from the adaptation of the autonomic nervous system to exercise training [32,33]. In this study, the decrease in the resting heart rate and the systemic norepinephrine concentration (Table 1) following URT may in part explain the reduction in AIx. Furthermore, previous studies imply that an increase in muscular strength after exercise training is associated with a decrease in central artery stiffness. Fahs et al. reported that adults who have higher muscular strength present lower central artery stiffness; particularly, those who have higher upper-limb muscular strength tend to have lower central artery stiffness [34]. In response to 8 weeks of URT, 1 RM of upper-limb resistance exercises was improved with a simultaneous increase in arm LBM in this study. The increase in muscular strength accompanying muscle hypertrophy may in part account for AIx reduction after URT. Change in AIx after the resistance exercise was associated with change in serum triglyceride levels. Blood triglyceride concentration measured after overnight fasting is used as a traditional marker of CVD risk. Considering both that endothelial dysfunction is a strong early marker to predict future CVD risk and that vascular endothelial dysfunction is closely related to serum triglyceride concentration, a decrease in serum triglyceride concentration after resistance training may contribute to a decrease in central artery stiffness via enhanced vascular endothelial function [35].

ArmPWV, a measure of peripheral artery stiffness in this study, showed a tendency to decrease in response to URT, although this tendency was not statistically significant. This result is different from the results of previous studies. Okamoto et al. reported that 8 weeks of single arm-curl resistance exercise increased baPWV, which is another measure of peripheral artery stiffness reflecting mainly lower-limb artery stiffness, in young women [36]. Similarly, 10 weeks of URT increased baPWV in young adults [37]. However, LRT did not influence baPWV in young adults and did not show any negative effects on AorPWV, the gold standard measure of central artery stiffness, in older adults [37,38]. The acute effects of one bout of resistance exercise on arterial stiffness can be different based on the exercising limbs. Li et al. reported that one bout of upper-limb resistance exercise increased baPWV, but lower-limb resistance exercise did not increase central artery stiffness in young men [39]. Similarly, in young adults, one bout of lower-limb resistance exercise did not show any negative effect on central artery stiffness [40]. In previous findings, the effects of resistance exercise on arterial stiffness were different according to the participant's age, gender, exercising limbs, training duration, and vascular beds measured for arterial stiffness assessment. Additionally, it is speculated that any difference in the effect of resistance exercise on peripheral artery stiffness between this study and the previous findings may be due to the difference in the employed methodologies—ArmPWV vs. baPWV.

No improvement was noted in the LegPWV following the 8-week LRT. However, for both resistance training groups (URT and LRT), the change in leg LBM had a significant relationship with the change in LegPWV. Resistance training can reduce peripheral artery stiffness not only by decreasing the trained peripheral artery tone at rest [41,42] but also by local vasodilation induced by increased circulating metabolites generated from resistance training [43]. Thus, this result suggests that improved vascular endothelial function after limb-specific resistance training via both local and systemic biochemical environment change may lead to enhanced peripheral artery stiffness even in relatively healthier young adults. Unfortunately, the related physiological mechanism could not be demonstrated because vascular endothelial function measures were not performed in this study.

Resting norepinephrine concentration significantly decreased and resting epinephrine concentration showed a tendency to decrease in all three groups following the 8 weeks of intervention. In particular, the reduction of systemic norepinephrine level in CON is likely associated with the impact of seasonal ambient temperature variations on the autonomic nervous system. The plasma catecholamine level in the cold ambient temperature is higher than that in the warm outside temperature, which is likely related to the increased cardiovascular morbidity and mortality in winter [44–49]. In this study, blood collection pre- and post-intervention was performed in March and July in 2017. The average ambient temperatures at Incheon, Korea during March and July in 2017 were 5.8 and 25.8 °C, respectively. It is speculated that the seasonal difference of ambient temperature might cause the significant difference in resting norepinephrine concentration between pre- and post-intervention.

This study has limitations that should be considered when interpreting major findings. The study was conducted with a relatively small number of healthy young adults. Thus, the research results cannot be generalized and applied to other populations with different biological or clinical conditions. In this study, the number of study participants by gender was not able to secure statistical power, making it impossible to further analyze gender differences. This study mainly analyzed functional changes, and there was a limit to the analysis of physiological mechanisms. In the future, large-scale functional and mechanistic research studies in which a sufficient number of men and women of various ages and health conditions participate are needed.

5. Conclusions

URT reduces pulse wave reflection, an index of arterial stiffness, and may be beneficial in decreasing local peripheral artery stiffness even in healthy young adults. Decreased serum triglyceride concentration and increased regional muscle mass in response to resistance training may contribute to the reduction of pulse wave reflection and peripheral artery stiffness in young individuals. These findings have clinical implications for the improvement of cardiovascular function and the prevention and management of cardiovascular disease for individuals with limitations in lower-limb movement or activity, such as injured veterans and disabled persons.

Author Contributions: Conceptualization, M.K. and M.-H.H.; methodology, M.K., R.L. and M.-H.H.; formal analysis, M.K., N.K. and M.-H.H.; investigation, M.K. and R.L.; resources, M.-H.H.; data curation, N.K. and M.-H.H.; writing—original draft preparation, M.K.; writing—review and editing, R.L., N.K. and M.-H.H.; supervision, M.-H.H.; project administration, M.K. and M.-H.H.; funding acquisition, M.-H.H. All authors have read and agreed to the published version of the manuscript.

Funding: This research was funded by the Incheon National University Research Grant in 2016 to Moon-Hyon Hwang.

Institutional Review Board Statement: The study was conducted according to the guidelines of the Declaration of Helsinki and approved by the Institutional Review Board of Incheon National University (approval# 7007971-201612-004-01 and the study protocol was approved on 12 December 2016).

Informed Consent Statement: Informed consent was obtained from all subjects involved in the study.

Data Availability Statement: Not applicable.

Acknowledgments: We thank the study participants for their time and effort.

Conflicts of Interest: The authors declare no conflict of interest.

References

1. DeVan, A.E.; Anton, M.M.; Cook, J.N.; Neidre, D.B.; Cortez-Cooper, M.Y.; Tanaka, H. Acute effects of resistance exercise on arterial compliance. *J. Appl. Physiol.* **2005**, *98*, 2287–2291. [CrossRef]
2. Nichols, W.W.; Singh, B.M. Augmentation index as a measure of peripheral vascular disease state. *Curr. Opin. Cardiol.* **2002**, *17*, 543–551. [CrossRef] [PubMed]
3. O'Rourke, M. Arterial stiffness, systolic blood pressure, and logical treatment of arterial hypertension. *Hypertension* **1990**, *15*, 339–347. [CrossRef] [PubMed]
4. Tanaka, H.; DeSouza, C.A.; Seals, D.R. Absence of age-related increase in central arterial stiffness in physically active women. *Arterioscler. Thromb. Vasc. Biol.* **1998**, *18*, 127–132. [CrossRef] [PubMed]
5. Urbina, E.M.; Kieltkya, L.; Tsai, J.; Srinivasan, S.R.; Berenson, G.S. Impact of multiple cardiovascular risk factors on brachial artery distensibility in young adults: The Bogalusa Heart Study. *Am. J. Hypertens.* **2005**, *18*, 767–771. [CrossRef] [PubMed]
6. Moreau, K.L.; Donato, A.J.; Seals, D.R.; DeSouza, C.A.; Tanaka, H. Regular exercise, hormone replacement therapy and the age-related decline in carotid arterial compliance in healthy women. *Cardiovasc. Res.* **2003**, *57*, 861–868. [CrossRef]
7. Moreau, K.L.; Degarmo, R.; Langley, J.; McMahon, C.; Howley, E.T.; Bassett, D.R.; Thompson, D.L. Increasing daily walking lowers blood pressure in postmenopausal women. *Med. Sci. Sports Exerc.* **2001**, *33*, 1825–1831. [CrossRef] [PubMed]
8. Okamoto, T.; Masuhara, M.; Ikuta, K. Home-based resistance training improves arterial stiffness in healthy premenopausal women. *Eur. J. Appl. Physiol.* **2009**, *107*, 113–117. [CrossRef] [PubMed]
9. Okamoto, T.; Masuhara, M.; Ikuta, K. Low-intensity resistance training after high-intensity resistance training can prevent the increase of central arterial stiffness. *Int. J. Sports Med.* **2013**, *34*, 385–390. [CrossRef]
10. DeSouza, C.A.; Shapiro, L.F.; Clevenger, C.M.; Dinenno, F.A.; Monahan, K.D.; Tanaka, H.; Seals, D.R. Regular aerobic exercise prevents and restores age-related declines in endothelium-dependent vasodilation in healthy men. *Circulation* **2000**, *102*, 1351–1357. [CrossRef]
11. Hwang, M.-H.; Kim, S. Type 2 diabetes: Endothelial dysfunction and Exercise. *J. Exerc. Nutr. Biochem.* **2014**, *18*, 239–247. [CrossRef] [PubMed]
12. Jeon, K.; Lee, S.; Hwang, M.-H. Effects of combined circuit exercise on arterial stiffness in hypertensive postmenopausal women: A local public center-based pilot study. *Menopause* **2018**, *25*, 1442–1447. [CrossRef]
13. Garber, C.E.; Blissmer, B.; Deschenes, M.R.; Franklin, B.A.; Lamonte, M.J.; Lee, I.M.; Nieman, D.C.; Swain, D.P. Quantity and quality of exercise for developing and maintaining cardiorespiratory, musculoskeletal, and neuromotor fitness in apparently healthy adults: Guidance for prescribing exercise. *Med. Sci. Sports Exerc.* **2011**, *43*, 1334–1359. [CrossRef] [PubMed]
14. Sugawara, J.; Otsuki, T.; Tanabe, T.; Hayashi, K.; Maeda, S.; Matsuda, M. Physical Activity Duration, Intensity, and Arterial Stiffening in Postmenopausal Women. *Am. J. Hypertens.* **2006**, *19*, 1032–1036. [CrossRef] [PubMed]
15. Tanaka, H.; Dinenno, F.A.; Monahan, K.D.; Clevenger, C.M.; DeSouza, C.A.; Seals, D.R. Aging, habitual exercise, and dynamic arterial compliance. *Circulation* **2000**, *102*, 1270–1275. [CrossRef]
16. Pollock, M.L.; Franklin, B.A.; Balady, G.J.; Chaitman, B.R.; Fleg, J.L.; Fletcher, B.; Limacher, M.C.; Pina, I.L.; Stein, R.A.; Williams, M.; et al. Resistance exercise in individuals with and without cardiovascular disease: Benefit, rationale, safety, and prescription. 2000, 8721, 1591–1597. *Circulation* **2020**, *101*, 828–833.
17. Haskell, W.L.; Lee, I.M.; Pate, R.R.; Powell, K.E.; Blair, S.N.; Franklin, B.A.; Macera, C.A.; Heath, G.W.; Thompson, P.D.; Bauman, A. Physical activity and public health: Updated recommendation for adults from the American College of Sports Medicine and the American Heart Association. *Circulation* **2007**, *116*, 1081–1093. [CrossRef]
18. Miyachi, M.; Donato, A.J.; Yamamoto, K.; Takahashi, K.; Gates, P.E.; Moreau, K.L.; Tanaka, H. Greater age-related reductions in central arterial compliance in resistance-trained men. *Hypertension* **2003**, *41*, 130–135. [CrossRef] [PubMed]
19. Cortez-Cooper, M.Y.; DeVan, A.E.; Anton, M.M.; Farrar, R.P.; Beckwith, K.A.; Todd, J.S.; Tanaka, H. Effects of high intensity resistance training on arterial stiffness and wave reflection in women. *Am. J. Hypertens.* **2005**, *18*, 930–934. [CrossRef]
20. Collier, S.R.; Kanaley, J.A.; Carhart, R.; Frechette, V.; Tobin, M.M.; Hall, A.K.; Luckenbaugh, A.N.; Fernhall, B. Effect of 4 weeks of aerobic or resistance exercise training on arterial stiffness, blood flow and blood pressure in pre- and stage-1 hypertensives. *J. Hum. Hypertens.* **2008**, *22*, 678–686. [CrossRef]
21. Kawano, H.; Tanaka, H.; Miyachi, M. Resistance training and arterial compliance keeping the benefits while minimizing the stiffening. *J. Hypertens.* **2006**, *24*, 1753–1759. [CrossRef]
22. Okamoto, T.; Masuhara, M.; Ikuta, K. Effect of low-intensity resistance training on arterial function. *Eur. J. Appl. Physiol.* **2011**, *111*, 743–748. [CrossRef] [PubMed]
23. Okamoto, T.; Min, S.; Sakamaki-Sunaga, M. Arterial compliance and stiffness following low-intensity resistance exercise. *Eur. J. Appl. Physiol.* **2014**, *114*, 235–241. [CrossRef] [PubMed]
24. Yoshizawa, M.; Maeda, S.; Miyaki, A.; Misono, M.; Choi, Y.; Shimojo, N.; Ajisaka, R.; Tanaka, H. Additive beneficial effects of lactotripeptides and aerobic exercise on arterial compliance in postmenopausal women. *Am. J. Physiol. Heart Circ. Physiol.* **2009**, *297*, H1899–H1903. [CrossRef]
25. Pauca, A.L.; O'Rourke, M.F.; Kon, N.D. Prospective evaluation of a method for estimating ascending aortic pressure from the radial artery pressure waveform. *Hypertension* **2001**, *38*, 932–937. [CrossRef]
26. Adji, A.; Hirata, K.; Hoegler, S.; O'Rourke, M.F. Noninvasive Pulse Waveform Analysis in Clinical Trials: Similarity of Two Methods for Calculating Aortic Systolic Pressure. *Am. J. Hypertens.* **2007**, *20*, 917–922. [CrossRef]

27. O'Rourke, M.F.; Hashimoto, J. Pressure pulse waveform analysis in critical care. *Crit. Care Med.* **2006**, *34*, 1569–1570. [CrossRef]
28. Hwang, M.-H.; Yoo, J.K.; Kim, H.K.; Hwang, C.L.; Mackay, K.; Hemstreet, O.; Nichols, W.W.; Christou, D.D. Validity and reliability of aortic pulse wave velocity and augmentation index determined by the new cuff-based SphygmoCor Xcel. *J. Hum. Hypertens.* **2014**, *28*, 475–481. [CrossRef] [PubMed]
29. Laurent, S.; Cockcroft, J.; Van Bortel, L.; Boutouyrie, P.; Giannattasio, C.; Hayoz, D.; Pannier, B.; Vlachopoulos, C.; Wilkinson, I.; Struijker-Boudier, H. Expert consensus document on arterial stiffness: Methodological issues and clinical applications. *Eur. Heart J.* **2006**, *27*, 2588–2605. [CrossRef] [PubMed]
30. LeSuer, D.A.; McCormick, J.H.; Mayhew, J.L.; Wasserstein, R.L.; Arnold, M.D. The accuracy of prediction equations for estimating 1-RM performance in the bench press, squat, and deadlift. *J. Strength Cond. Res.* **1997**, *11*, 211–213.
31. Ray, C.A.; Carrasco, D.I. Isometric handgrip training reduces arterial pressure at rest without changes in sympathetic nerve activity. *Am. J. Physiol. Heart Circ. Physiol.* **2000**, *279*, H245–H249. [CrossRef]
32. Tartière, J.M.; Logeart, D.; Safar, M.E.; Cohen-Solal, A. Interaction between pulse wave velocity, augmentation index, pulse pressure and left ventricular function in chronic heart failure. *J. Hum. Hypertens.* **2006**, *20*, 213–219. [CrossRef]
33. Wilkinson, I.B.; Franklin, S.S.; Cockcroft, J.R. Nitric Oxide and the Regulation of Large Artery Stiffness. *Hypertension* **2004**, *44*, 112–116. [CrossRef] [PubMed]
34. Fahs, C.A.; Heffernan, K.S.; Ranadive, S.; Jae, S.Y.; Fernhall, B. Muscular strength is inversely associated with aortic stiffness in young men. *Med. Sci. Sports Exerc.* **2010**, *42*, 1619–1624. [CrossRef] [PubMed]
35. Jagla, A.; Schrezenmeir, J. Postprandial triglycerides and endothelial function. *Exp. Clin. Endocrinol. Diabetes* **2001**, *109*, 533–547. [CrossRef] [PubMed]
36. Okamoto, T.; Masuhara, M.; Ikuta, K. Effects of eccentric and concentric resistance training on arterial stiffness. *J. Hum. Hypertens.* **2006**, *20*, 348–354. [CrossRef] [PubMed]
37. Okamoto, T.; Masuhara, M.; Ikuta, K. Upper but not lower limb resistance training increases arterial stiffness in humans. *Eur. J. Appl. Physiol.* **2009**, *107*, 127–134. [CrossRef]
38. Maeda, S.; Otsuki, T.; Iemitsu, M.; Kamioka, M.; Sugawara, J.; Kuno, S.; Ajisaka, R.; Tanaka, H. Effects of leg resistance training on arterial function in older men. *Br. J. Sports Med.* **2006**, *40*, 867–869. [CrossRef] [PubMed]
39. Li, Y.; Bopp, M.; Botta, F.; Nussbaumer, M.; Schäfer, J.; Roth, R.; Schmidt-Trucksäss, A.; Hanssen, H. Lower Body vs. Upper Body Resistance Training and Arterial Stiffness in Young Men. *Int. J. Sports Med.* **2015**, *36*, 960–967. [CrossRef]
40. Heffernan, K.S.; Rossow, L.; Jae, S.Y.; Shokunbi, H.G.; Gibson, E.M.; Fernhall, B. Effect of single-leg resistance exercise on regional arterial stiffness. *Eur. J. Appl. Physiol.* **2006**, *98*, 185–190. [CrossRef]
41. Bank, A.J.; Kaiser, D.R. Smooth muscle relaxation: Effects on arterial compliance, distensibility, elastic modulus, and pulse wave velocity. *Hypertension* **1998**, *32*, 356–359. [CrossRef]
42. Kingwell, B.A.; Berry, K.L.; Cameron, J.D.; Jennings, G.L.; Dart, A.M. Arterial compliance increases after moderate-intensity cycling. *Am. J. Physiol. Circ. Physiol.* **1997**, *42*, H2186–H2191. [CrossRef]
43. Green, D.J.; O'Driscoll, G.; Blanksby, B.A.; Taylor, R.R. Control of skeletal muscle blood flow during dynamic exercise. *Sport. Med.* **1996**, *21*, 119–146. [CrossRef] [PubMed]
44. Radke, K.J.; Izzo, J.L. Seasonal variation in haemodynamics and blood pressure-regulating hormones. *J. Hum. Hypertens.* **2010**, *24*, 410–416. [CrossRef]
45. Kruse, H.J.; Wieczorek, I.; Hecker, H.; Creutzig, A.; Schellong, S.M. Seasonal variation of endothelin-1, angiotensin II, and plasma catecholamines and their relation to outside temperature. *J. Lab. Clin. Med.* **2002**, *140*, 236–241. [CrossRef]
46. Hiramatsu, K.; Yamada, T.; Katakura, M. Acute effects of cold on blood pressure, renin-angiotensin-aldosterone system, catecholamines and adrenal steroids in man. *Clin. Exp. Pharmacol. Physiol.* **1984**, *11*, 171–179. [CrossRef] [PubMed]
47. Healy, J.D. Excess winter mortality in Europe: A cross country analysis identifying key risk factors. *J. Epidemiol. Community Health* **2003**, *57*, 784–789. [CrossRef] [PubMed]
48. Turner, L.R.; Barnett, A.G.; Connell, D.; Tonga, S. Ambient temperature and cardiorespiratory morbidity: A systematic review and meta-analysis. *Epidemiology* **2012**, *23*, 594–606. [CrossRef]
49. Myint, P.K.; Vowler, S.L.; Woodhouse, P.R.; Redmayne, O.; Fulcher, R.A. Winter excess in hospital admissions, in-patient mortality and length of acute hospital stay in stroke: A hospital database study over six seasonal years in Nirfolk, UK. *Neuroepidemiology* **2007**, *28*, 79–85. [CrossRef]

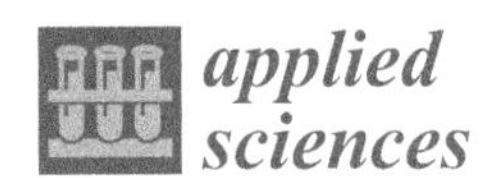

MDPI

Article

Effects of Core Stabilization Exercise Programs on Changes in Erector Spinae Contractile Properties and Isokinetic Muscle Function of Adult Females with a Sedentary Lifestyle

Hyungwoo Lee [1,2], Chanki Kim [1,2], Seungho An [1,2] and Kyoungkyu Jeon [2,3,4,5,*]

1 Department of Human Movement Science, Incheon National University, 119 Academy-ro, Yeonsu-gu, Incheon 22012, Korea; guddn318@inu.ac.kr (H.L.); kimchangi960430@gmail.com (C.K.); hshsh96@gmail.com (S.A.)
2 Functional Rehabilitation Biomechanics Laboratory, Incheon National University, 119 Academy-ro, Yeonsu-gu, Incheon 22012, Korea
3 Division of Sport Science, Incheon National University, 119 Academy-ro, Yeonsu-gu, Incheon 22012, Korea
4 Sport Science Institute, Incheon National University, 119 Academy-ro, Yeonsu-gu, Incheon 22012, Korea
5 Health Promotion Center, Incheon National University, 119 Academy-ro, Yeonsu-gu, Incheon 22012, Korea
* Correspondence: jeonkay@inu.ac.kr

Abstract: This study aimed to investigate the effect of core stabilization exercises on the contractile properties and isokinetic muscle function of adult females with a sedentary lifestyle. We enrolled 105 adult females. Tensiomyography was performed on the erector spinae, and the isokinetic muscular functional test was performed on the trunk at an angular velocity of 60°/s and 90°/s. All participants performed the exercise for 60 min per day, 3 times a week, for 7 weeks. A Wilcoxon signed-rank test was performed at a significance level of 0.05. Tensiomyography (TMG) of the erector spinae revealed no significant post-exercise change in the contraction time; however, there was a significant post-exercise increase in the maximum radial displacement and mean velocity until 90% of the TMG was displaced. Additionally, the isokinetic muscular functional test of the trunk revealed a significant post-exercise increase in almost all variables. Our findings demonstrated that the core stabilization exercise reduced stiffness in the erector spinae, increased the velocity of erector spinae contraction, and effectively improved the isokinetic muscular function of the trunk.

Keywords: sedentary behavior; core stabilization training; neuromuscular properties; muscle function

Citation: Lee, H.; Kim, C.; An, S.; Jeon, K. Effects of Core Stabilization Exercise Programs on Changes in Erector Spinae Contractile Properties and Isokinetic Muscle Function of Adult Females with a Sedentary Lifestyle. *Appl. Sci.* **2022**, *12*, 2501. https://doi.org/10.3390/app12052501

Academic Editor: Jesús García Pallarés

Received: 24 January 2022
Accepted: 25 February 2022
Published: 28 February 2022

1. Introduction

There have been rapid changes in the physical, economic, and social environment in which modern-day people perform activities, which has contributed to a distinct decrease in physical activities [1]. The World Health Organization (WHO) recommends at least either 150 or 75 min of moderate- or high-intensity physical activity, respectively, or both to prevent reductions in physical activity levels [2]. The COVID-19 pandemic has caused many changes in our daily life, one of those is that physical activity level has decreased, whereas sedentary lifestyles have increased [3]. The resulting lack of physical activity and increasingly sedentary lifestyle can cause numerous physical problems; further, maintaining a sedentary lifestyle for >4 h a day can threaten health [4,5].

Functional decline caused by decreased physical activity, including muscle imbalance, muscle weakness, and loss of flexibility, can cause chronic musculoskeletal disorders [6]. Low-back pain is strongly associated with a sedentary lifestyle [7]; specifically, a more sedentary lifestyle is an independent risk factor for musculoskeletal disorders [8]. Further, a sedentary lifestyle is a risk factor for low-back pain since it can cause muscle fatigue, due to continued core muscle contractions, increased intradiscal loads, and the weakening of the posterior lumbar structure [9,10]. Kett et al. [8,11] reported increased lumbar muscle stiffness, as measured by an indentometer, after 4.5 h of sedentary work. Moreover, musculoskeletal disorders in the lower back may be caused by increased sedentary patterns since they increase muscle tension and sustain a shortened state in the lumbar region [8,11]. Additionally, a decreased spinal stabilization function due to the lumbar muscle weakening is a major cause of low-back pain [12,13]. Patients with low-back pain due to spinal instability have muscle tissue tension and damage due to the weakening of their lumbar extensors; accordingly, >85% of the total population experiences chronic low-back pain [14–16]. Previous studies have reported that women are more likely to be exposed to risk factors such as improper static posture [17], and the prevalence of low-back pain was higher in women than in men [18]. In women, it has been reported that there is a tendency to present worse and more persistent pain symptoms [19]. As aforementioned, increased tension and weakness in the trunk extensor resulting from a sedentary lifestyle can result in an increased incidence of low-back pain. Therefore, trunk-strengthening exercises are essential for reducing the incidence of low-back pain [9,11,14].

Patil and Mahajan [20] recently reported a significant improvement in core stability after prescribing a regular plank exercise for 6 weeks to 50 dentists who performed sedentary work for long hours. In a study on patients with non-specific low-back pain, Narouei et al. [21] reported that regular core stabilization exercise for 4 weeks could effectively increase muscle contractile thickness and reduce pain. Moreover, a study using a Swiss ball for 8 weeks reported a significant increase in core muscle activity after core stabilization exercises [22]. This broad range of benefits resulting from core stabilization can enhance exercise ability, prevent injuries, and alleviate low-back pain, which facilitates proper load balancing within the kinetic chain involving the spine and pelvis [23]. Therefore, systematic exercises for ensuring core stability are paramount for preventing a deterioration in trunk muscle function and low-back pain. However, previous studies on sedentary lifestyles have mostly focused on the physiological effects, including cardiovascular and metabolic effects, of lacking physical activities [24–27]. Moreover, few studies have applied systematic trunk exercise interventions for alleviating deteriorations in trunk muscle functions due to a sedentary lifestyle, with a concomitant assessment of the mechanical and neuromuscular properties of trunk muscles and the isokinetic muscle functions of the lumbar spine. Given the increasing amount of time spent sitting by modern-day people, there is a need for studies on appropriate exercise interventions for trunk stabilization that analyze the isokinetic muscle function of the lumbar spine and the mechanical and neuromuscular properties of trunk muscles.

Based on previous studies, muscle fatigue tends to decrease the time it takes to contract 10 to 90% of the maximum contractile displacement (contraction time (Tc)) [28]. With the strengthening of the trunk muscles through exercise, Tc is expected to increase due to the reduction in muscle fatigue. The results of a previous study analyzing the effect of the 3D moving platform exercise for 8 weeks did not show statistical significance, but based on the study results showing an increase in the maximum radial displacement (Dm) of the muscle, Dm is expected to increase through exercise [29]. In addition, based on previous studies, core stabilization exercise increases neuromuscular control by improving the sensory receptors and motor control of the core muscle [23]. Therefore, Vc90 is expected to increase through core stabilization exercise. Additionally, based on a previous study where the isokinetic muscle function of the lumbar region improved after 12 weeks of lumbar stabilization exercise [30], the isokinetic muscle function of the trunk will be improved through core stabilization exercise.

Therefore, the central purpose of this study is to propose basic data for facilitating the development of an effective core stabilization exercise program for preventing musculoskeletal disorders caused by a lengthy sedentary lifestyle. Specifically, we aimed to determine the effects of a 7-week core stabilization exercise program on the mechanical and neuromuscular properties of the erector spinae, including muscle stiffness, contraction velocity, contractile response, maximum displacement, and the isokinetic muscle function of the trunk in adult females with sedentary work patterns.

2. Materials and Methods

2.1. Design and Participants

A single group crossover design was employed for this study. We included 105 female office workers aged ≥ 20 years who did not perform regular exercise for the past 6 months, did not meet the WHO-recommended physical activity levels, and performed at least 7 h of sedentary work per day. We excluded participants with a history of surgery or any musculoskeletal or neurological disorder within the past 3 months. To ensure we included participants without problems performing physical activities, we only selected participants who reported lacking limitations in activities of daily living due to a current health problem or physical or mental disability. This study was approved by the Institutional Review Board of the Incheon National University (INUIRB No. 7007971-202012-003A). The participants provided informed consent after receiving sufficient explanations regarding the study contents and procedures. The specific demographic information and physical activity are shown in Table 1.

Table 1. Demographic information and physical activity of participants.

	Variables	Values
Participants	N	105
	Age (years)	30.99 ± 10.85
	Weight (kg)	57.79 ± 10.44
	Height (cm)	159.99 ± 15.03
Physical Activity	Vigorous intensity (day/week)	0.29 ± 15.03
	Vigorous intensity (min/day)	10.19 ± 19.65
	Moderate intensity (day/week)	0.66 ± 0.90
	Moderate intensity (min/day)	18.35 ± 29.80
	Sedentary time (min/day)	469.71 ± 45.16

Note. Data are mean ± standard deviation.

2.2. Procedures

2.2.1. Tensiomyography

A tensiomyography (TMG-100 System electrostimulator, Slovenia), which is a device used to analyze the contractile properties of muscles, was used to assess the mechanical and neuromuscular properties of the erector spinae (Figure 1). Since Domaszewski et al. [31] reported that caffeine intake may affect muscle contraction time and displacement, the participants were asked to refrain from caffeine intake for 24 h before the measurement. Moreover, the participants were requested to avoid exercise and fascia treatment that could cause fatigue for 48 h before the measurement. Measurements were performed after enough rest to ensure that the erector spinae muscle was maintained in a relaxed state. Further, measurements were performed in a static position to minimize variability of the TMG sensor position. To ensure accurate measurement with minimal lumbar lordosis, a wedge cushion was placed on the ankles and the anterior superior iliac spine (ASIS) in a prone position; moreover, a pad was placed on the ankles to maintain knee flexion at approximately 5°. Subsequently, we examined the proximal region of the erector spinae muscle. The digital displacement sensor (GK40, Ljubljana, Slovenia) was vertically placed 5 cm above the posterior superior iliac spine (PSIS), with a maximum radial displacement (Dm) of 15 mm. The distance between the electrode pads was maintained at 5 cm. A single electrical stimulus was started at 20 mA, followed by 20-mA increments. Measurements were gradually obtained until maximum displacement appeared. A 15 s rest period was allowed between measurements to minimize muscle fatigue; further, all measurements were conducted from right to left.

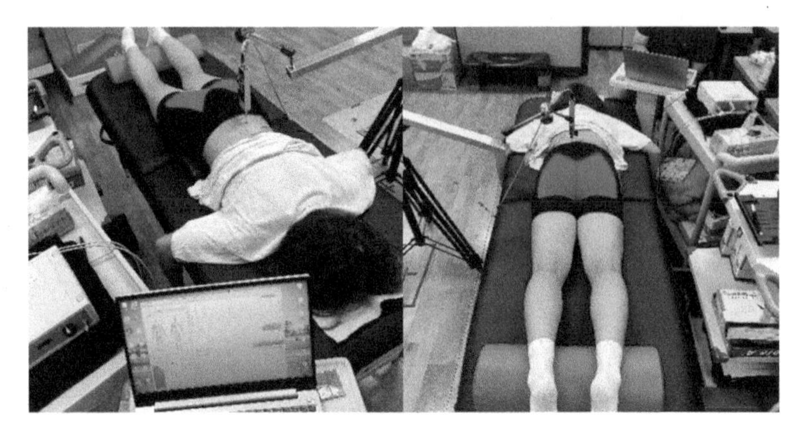

Figure 1. Tensiomyography device and appropriate prone position.

2.2.2. Isokinetic Muscle–Joint Function Test

We performed isokinetic muscle–joint function tests (Humac Norm Testing and Rehabilitation, CSMi Medical & Solution, Stoughton, MA, USA) on the trunk (Figure 2). The participants performed sufficient warm-up exercises, such as dynamic stretching for trunk flexion and extension, before the measurements to prevent injury. A trunk adapter was connected to the dynamometer of the test equipment; additionally, the footpad was adjusted by aligning the anatomical vertical axis with the equipment axis. To generate maximum muscle strength during trunk flexion and extension, the lower extremities were fixed using popliteal, femoral, tibial, and pelvic belts. To minimize interference from nearby joint movements, the upper extremities were fixed using a shoulder pad at the inferior scapular angle. The joint range of motion (ROM) was restricted by setting the ROM to the maximum flexion and extension possible without pain, to prevent injury resulting from excessive flexion or extension. Subsequently, a preliminary exercise was performed to ensure familiarity with the measurement equipment. A 2-min rest period was allowed to minimize muscle fatigue between measurements; further, measurements were performed 5 and 15 times at an angular velocity of 60°/s and 90°/s, respectively.

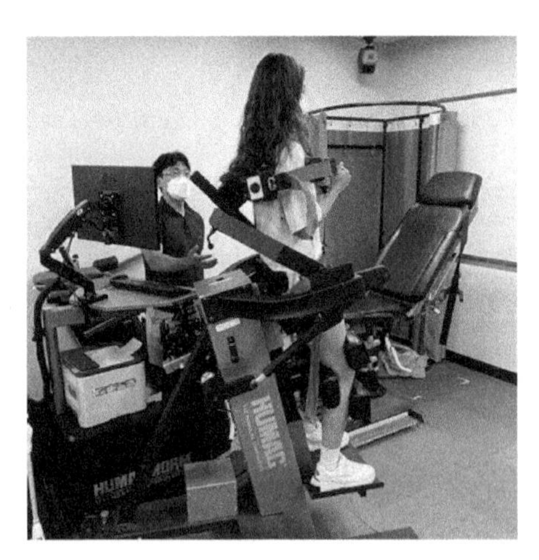

Figure 2. Humac Norm Testing and Rehabilitation device with trunk adapt.

2.3. Core Stabilization Exercise Program

The exercise program comprised warm-up, main, and cool-down exercises. Warm-up and cool-down exercises were performed for 10 min each using a foam roller to allow self-fascia relaxation as well as static and dynamic stretching, with the intensity set at a pain-free range. The workout mostly comprised core stabilization exercises involving 3 60-min exercise sessions per week. The main exercise focused on muscles around the lower back and hips that contribute to core stabilization, for improved trunk muscle strength and endurance, coordination, proprioceptive function, and stability. Based on previous studies, the core stabilization exercise programs comprised traditional core exercises, including bracing, hollowing to activate the abdominal wall musculature, bird dog, plank, back extensions, and hip bridge, as well as the trunk twist hip bridge to activate the lumbar paraspinals [23,32] (Table 2). Thabet et al. [32] prescribed an exercise intervention to postpartum women that comprised 3 sets of 20 repetitions, with 5 s of contraction and 10 s of relaxation. Since we included healthy adult females, they were requested to perform 5 s of contraction and 5 s of relaxation for more intense exercise.

Table 2. Core stabilization intervention program.

Classification	Exercise Type	Exercise	Intensity	Time
Warm-up	Self-myofascial release (Foam roller)	Quadriceps rolling Hamstring rolling Gluteus rolling Back (lower and upper) rolling	Pain-free range 20 s/1 set Total 3 sets	10 min
	Stretching (Static and Dynamic)	Quadriceps stretching Hamstring stretching Gluteus stretching Erector spinae stretching Cat-camel stretching Hip flexion and extension		
Main Exercise	Core stabilization exercise	Bracing and Hollowing Plank (side and prone) Hip Bridge Back Extension Bird dog Trunk Twist	1 rep (5 s contraction 5 s relaxation) 20 reps/1 set Total 3 sets	40 min
Cool-down	Self-myofascial release (Foam roller)	Quadriceps rolling Hamstring rolling Gluteus rolling Back (lower and upper) rolling	Pain-free range 20 s/1 set Total 3 sets	10 min
	Stretching (Static and Dynamic)	Quadriceps stretching Hamstring stretching Gluteus stretching Erector spinae stretching Cat-camel stretching Hip flexion and extension		

2.4. Data Analysis

2.4.1. Analysis of Mechanical and Neuromuscular Properties of Muscle

To analyze the mechanical and neuromuscular properties, we applied a range of 0.91–0.99 for Dm, which indicates the maximum contractile displacement as the variable with the highest measure-remeasure and intra-rater reliability indices, and a range of 0.70–0.98 for contraction time (Tc), which is the time required for contraction to reach 10–90% of the maximum contractile displacement [33,34]. Since Tc could be influenced by the Dm magnitude, we calculated the mean velocity until 90% Dm (Vc90), using the equation $Vc90 = \frac{Dm*0.9}{Tc+Td}$ to assess muscle contraction velocity [35,36]. Bilateral values of all measured variables were summed, and the mean values were calculated.

2.4.2. Analysis of Isokinetic Muscle Function of Trunk

The maximum muscle strength of the flexor and extensor muscles at all angular velocities was analyzed. The absolute muscle strength was divided by the bodyweight of each participant to derive relative muscle strength. Additionally, to assess the flexor and extensor muscle balance in the trunk, we used the muscle strength ratio to analyze the isokinetic muscle function of the trunk.

2.5. Statistical Processing

All statistical analyses were performed using SPSS 26.0 (IBM, Chicago, IL, USA). The mean and standard deviation of each variable was calculated. The Kolmogorov-Smirnov test showed that the data was not normally distributed. The Wilcoxon signed-rank test was used for within-group comparisons of pre- and post-intervention measurements. Statistical significance was set at $p < 0.05$.

3. Results

3.1. Analysis of Mechanical and Neuromuscular Properties of the Erector Spinae

There was a significant post-exercise change in Dm ($z = -3.998$; $p < 0.001$) and Vc90 ($z = -3.889$; $p < 0.001$), but not Tc ($z = -1.143$; $p = 0.253$) (Table 3).

Table 3. Results of tensiomyography of erector spinae of the participants.

Variables	Pre	Post	z	p
Tc (ms)	16.37 ± 3.98	16.38 ± 3.44	−1.143	0.253
Dm (mm)	2.49 ± 1.32	2.87 ± 1.14	−3.998	<0.001 ***
Vc90 (mm/ms)	0.06 ± 0.04	0.07 ± 0.03	−3.889	<0.001 ***

Note. Data are mean ± standard deviation, *** $p < 0.001$. Abbreviations: Tc, contraction time; Dm, Maximum radial displacement; Vc90, Mean velocity until 90%.

3.2. Analysis of Isokinetic Muscle Function of Trunk

At an angular velocity of 60°/s, there was a significant post-exercise change in the maximum ($z = -6.605$; $p < 0.001$) and relative muscle strength per bodyweight of the extensor ($z = -6.681$; $p < 0.001$), but there was not a significant post-exercise change for the flexor ($z = -0.686$; $p = 0.493$, $z = -0.887$; $p = 0.375$) (Table 4).

Table 4. Results for isokinetic muscle function of trunk.

	Variables		Pre	Post	z	p
60°/s	Flexor	PT (Nm)	132.19 ± 35.39	135.61 ± 29.74	−0.686	0.493
		PT (%BW)	227.52 ± 49.23	235.01 ± 37.99	−0.887	0.375
	Extensor	PT (Nm)	101.54 ± 37.79	118.92 ± 34.66	−6.605	<0.001 ***
		PT (%BW)	174.21 ± 57.58	206.11 ± 55.59	−6.681	<0.001 ***
	Ratio		139.43 ± 38.16	120.72 ± 31.86	−5.424	<0.001 ***
90°/s	Flexor	PT (Nm)	130.25 ± 34.65	133.55 ± 31.24	−1.461	0.144
		PT (%BW)	224.20 ± 46.92	232.03 ± 41.68	−1.950	0.051
	Extensor	PT (Nm)	88.55 ± 31.71	106.83 ± 30.75	−7.218	<0.001 ***
		PT (%BW)	152.30 ± 48.66	183.65 ± 46.55	−7.232	<0.001 ***
	Ratio		159.21 ± 52.48	132.07 ± 31.52	−6.285	<0.001 ***

Note. Data are mean ± standard deviation, *** $p < 0.001$. Abbreviations: PT, Peak torque; BW, Body weight.

At an angular velocity of 90°/s, there was no significant post-exercise change in the maximum and relative muscle strength ($z = -1.461$; $p = 0.144$, $z = -1.950$; $p = 0.051$) of the flexor muscle (Table 4). However, there was a significant post-exercise change in the maximum and relative muscle strength per bodyweight of the extensor muscle ($z = -7.218$; $p < 0.001$, $z = -7.232$; $p < 0.001$).

Regarding the muscle strength ratio, measurements at an angular velocity of 60°/s ($z = -5.424$; $p < 0.001$) and 90°/s ($z = -6.285$; $p < 0.001$) showed significant differences (Table 4).

4. Discussion and Limitation

This study presented basic data for facilitating the development of an effective exercise intervention program for preventing musculoskeletal disorders caused by a lengthy sedentary lifestyle. We determined the effects of a 7-week core stabilization exercise program on the mechanical and neuromuscular properties of the erector spinae and the isokinetic muscle function of the trunk in adult females who perform ≥ 7 h of sedentary work per day.

Regarding the mechanical and neuromuscular properties of the erector spinae muscle, there was a significant post-exercise increase in the Dm and Vc90, but not Tc, values. Tc showed higher and lower values in type I and II muscle fibers, respectively; specifically, Tc has a strong correlation with type I muscle fibers [37,38]. Given the nature of the erector spinae muscle, type I muscle fibers, which have strong fatigue resistance, are more dominant than type IIa or IIx muscle fibers in maintaining lumbar stability through continued contraction [39,40]. Furthermore, it is difficult to convert type I muscle fibers into type IIa and type IIx muscle fibers through training [41]. Consistent with this evidence, we observed no significant post-exercise change in the Tc of the erector spinae muscle.

Consistent with our hypothesis, there was a significant post-exercise increase in Dm. Dm is considered a scale for muscle stiffness; specifically, it is negatively correlated with muscle stiffness [42–44]. A lengthy sedentary lifestyle causes microdamage and spasms in muscle connective tissue, which increases muscle stiffness by restricting muscle tissue microcirculation [45,46]. Moreover, muscle stiffness showed a strong positive correlation with isometric contraction [47]. Kett et al. [8] reported a significant increase in lumbar muscle stiffness after 4–5 h of sedentary work and a significantly reduced muscle stiffness after an 8 min roller massage. Because roller massages break down the cross-bridges between the actin and myosin filaments that were previously formed by the prolonged sitting period, muscle stiffness is significantly reduced. Moreover, the effect of relaxing muscle tension and reducing muscle stiffness owing to self-fascial relaxation using a foam roller is known to have long-term effects [48]. Muscle stiffness increases immediately after exercise, which is relieved with repeated exercise [49]. Accordingly, erector spinae stiffness was reduced in participants through repeated exercise and self-fascial relaxation using a foam roller. As a result, there was a post-exercise increase in Dm.

Consistent with our hypothesis, Vc90 showed a significant post-intervention increase. This suggests a post-exercise increase in the contraction velocity of the erector spinae muscle. Core stabilization exercise can effectively stimulate the sensory receptors and motor control of core muscles and increase neuromuscular control and stability [23], with a concomitant increase in the core muscle activation [21,50]. Specifically, Mannion et al. [51] reported that stabilization exercise for ≥3 weeks is required to activate the erector spinae muscle in patients with non-specific chronic low-back pain. Accordingly, there was a post-exercise increase in core muscle activation and neuromuscular control; specifically, TMG measurement revealed an increased contraction velocity through the activation of the erector spinae muscle. This indicated that core stabilization was achieved through enhanced muscle function, which allowed lumbar stabilization during activities of daily living and sports activities, while changing appropriately to maintain proper postural control [40,52].

Regarding the isokinetic muscle function of the trunk, there was no significant post-exercise change in maximum and relative flexor muscle strength at an angular velocity of

60°/s, as well as maximum and relative flexor muscle strength at an angular velocity of 90°/s. However, there was a significant post-exercise increase in other variables, including maximum and relative extensor muscle strength at an angular velocity of 60°/s and 90°/s. Moreover, there was a significant decrease in the muscle ratio (ratio of the flexor and extensor muscles of the trunk) at an angular velocity of 60°/s and 90°/s.

Our findings demonstrated that the core stabilization exercise program strengthens core muscles, which improves the balanced development of flexor and extensor muscles, as well as enhances the isokinetic muscle functions of the trunk, including muscle strength and endurance. Accordingly, core stabilization exercises could effectively increase muscle strength in the trunk and improve neuromuscular imbalance. Moreover, a 12-week core stabilization exercise program was found to improve the strength of the lumbar flexor and extensor muscles in primary school students with scoliosis [53]. Additionally, an 8-week core stabilization exercise program was found to significantly increase flexor and extensor muscle strength at an angular velocity of 60°/s and 90°/s in women with a sedentary lifestyle [54]. Furthermore, Sipaviciene et al. [30] reported a 12-week lumbar stabilization exercise program improved isokinetic muscle function of the trunk in patients with non-specific chronic low-back pain. As aforementioned, most studies have demonstrated that core stabilization exercise enhances core muscle strength. In addition, core stabilization exercise increases lumbar stability by strengthening the core flexor and extensor muscles, as well as the contractile and neuromuscular control functions [55]. Consistent with these previous findings, we observed a significant post-exercise decrease in the muscle strength ratio, which was effective for the balanced development of core muscles.

The core muscles represent the anatomical and functional center of the body and play a corset-like role in stabilizing the body and spine [56]. Weakened lumbar muscles cause deterioration of the spinal stabilization function, which can be a primary cause of low-back pain [12,13]. Conversely, strengthening core muscles enhances core stability and is crucially involved in performing activities of daily living or various other activities, as well as maintaining posture and balance [57,58]. Our core stabilization exercise program enhanced lumbar muscle function and strength, which can enhance core stability and prevent musculoskeletal disorders caused by a lengthy sedentary lifestyle.

This study suggests that the core stabilization exercise program may have a positive effect on muscle stiffness and contraction rates in the group with long-term sedentary lifestyles. In addition, tensiomyography can be used to clinically evaluate muscle contraction characteristics. Limitations of this study were that there was no control group and only healthy subjects were recruited. In future studies, it is necessary to further study the effect of the core stabilization exercise program by composing a control group and a low-back-pain group.

5. Conclusions

This study presented basic data for facilitating the development of an exercise program for preventing musculoskeletal disorders caused by a sedentary lifestyle, by analyzing the effects of core stabilization exercise on the muscle contraction properties of the erector spinae and changes in the isokinetic muscle function in adult females with a sedentary lifestyle. We found that the 7-week core stabilization exercise program could effectively reduce muscle stiffness in the erector spinae muscle; moreover, it increased contraction velocity through activation of the neuromuscular control of the erector spinae muscle, and effectively enhanced isokinetic muscle function of the trunk.

Author Contributions: Conceptualization, K.J.; methodology, K.J. and H.L.; software, H.L. and C.K.; validation, K.J. and H.L.; formal analysis, H.L. and S.A.; investigation, K.J., H.L., C.K. and S.A.; resources, K.J.; data curation, K.J. and H.L.; writing—original draft preparation, K.J., H.L. and C.K.; writing-review and editing, K.J. and H.L.; visualization, visualization; supervision, K.J.; project administration, K.J.; funding acquisition, K.J. All authors have read and agreed to the published version of the manuscript.

Funding: This work was supported by the Research Assistance Program (2021) of the Incheon National University.

Institutional Review Board Statement: This study was approved by the Institutional Review Board of the Incheon National University (INUIRB No. 7007971-202012-003A).

Informed Consent Statement: Informed consent was obtained from all participants involved in the study.

Data Availability Statement: Data are not publicly available due to privacy.

Acknowledgments: The authors would like to thank the participants for their time and commitment to this research.

Conflicts of Interest: The authors have no financial or personal relationships with other people or organizations that have inappropriately influenced this research.

References

1. Owen, N.; Healy, G.N.; Matthews, C.E.; Dunstan, D.W. Too Much Sitting: The Population-Health Science of Sedentary Behavior. *Exerc. Sport Sci. Rev.* **2010**, *38*, 105–113. [CrossRef] [PubMed]
2. Romero-Blanco, C.; Rodríguez-Almagro, J.; Onieva-Zafra, M.D.; Parra-Fernández, M.L.; Prado-Laguna, M.D.C.; Hernández-Martínez, A. Physical Activity and Sedentary Lifestyle in University Students: Changes during Confinement Due to the COVID-19 Pandemic. *Int. J. Environ. Res. Public Health* **2020**, *17*, 6567. [CrossRef] [PubMed]
3. Stockwell, S.; Trott, M.; Tully, M.; Shin, J.; Barnett, Y.; Butler, L.; McDermott, D.; Schuch, F.; Smith, L. Changes in physical activity and sedentary behaviours from before to during the COVID-19 pandemic lockdown: A systematic review. *BMJ Open Sport Exerc. Med.* **2021**, *7*, e000960. [CrossRef]
4. Pratt, M.; Varela, A.R.; Salvo, D.; Kohl, H.W., III; Ding, D. Attacking the pandemic of physical inactivity: What is holding us back? *Br. J. Sports Med.* **2020**, *54*, 760–762. [CrossRef] [PubMed]
5. Ozemek, C.; Lavie, C.J.; Rognmo, Ø. Global physical activity levels-Need for intervention. *Prog. Cardiovasc. Dis.* **2019**, *62*, 102–107. [CrossRef]
6. Heneweer, H.; Vanhees, L.; Picavet, H.S.J. Physical activity and low back pain: A U-shaped relation? *Pain* **2009**, *143*, 21–25. [CrossRef]
7. Moreno, M.A.; Catai, A.M.; Teodori, R.M.; Borges, B.L.A.; Cesar, M.d.C.; Silva, E.d. Effect of a muscle stretching program using the Global Postural Reeducation method on respiratory muscle strength and thoracoabdominal mobility of sedentary young males. *J. Bras. Pneumol.* **2007**, *33*, 679–686. [CrossRef]
8. Kett, A.R.; Sichting, F. Sedentary behaviour at work increases muscle stiffness of the back: Why roller massage has potential as an active break intervention. *Appl. Ergon.* **2020**, *82*, 102947. [CrossRef]
9. Cho, K.H.; Beom, J.W.; Lee, T.S.; Lim, J.H.; Lee, T.H.; Yuk, J.H. Trunk Muscles Strength as a Risk Factor for Nonspecific Low Back Pain: A Pilot Study. *Ann. Rehabil. Med.* **2014**, *38*, 234–240. [CrossRef]
10. Saiklang, P.; Puntumetakul, R.; Selfe, J.; Yeowell, G. An Evaluation of an Innovative Exercise to Relieve Chronic Low Back Pain in Sedentary Workers. *Hum. Factors* **2020**, 1–15. [CrossRef]
11. Kett, A.R.; Sichting, F.; Milani, T.L. The Effect of Sitting Posture and Postural Activity on Low Back Muscle Stiffness. *Biomechanics* **2021**, *1*, 214–224. [CrossRef]
12. Kuster, R.P.; Bauer, C.M.; Baumgartner, D. Is active sitting on a dynamic office chair controlled by the trunk muscles? *PLoS ONE* **2020**, *15*, e0242854. [CrossRef] [PubMed]
13. Mörl, F.; Bradl, I. Lumbar posture and muscular activity while sitting during office work. *J. Electromyogr. Kinesiol.* **2013**, *23*, 362–368. [CrossRef] [PubMed]
14. Park, J.H.; Seo, K.S.; Lee, S.U. Effect of Superimposed Electromyostimulation on Back Extensor Strengthening: A Pilot Study. *J. Strength Cond. Res.* **2016**, *30*, 2470–2475. [CrossRef]
15. Hanna, F.; Daas, R.N.; El-Shareif, T.J.; Al-Marridi, H.H.; Al-Rojoub, Z.M.; Adegboye, O.A. The Relationship Between Sedentary Behavior, Back Pain, and Psychosocial Correlates Among University Employees. *Front. Public Health* **2019**, *7*, 80. [CrossRef]
16. Nowotny, A.H.; Calderon, M.G.; de Souza, P.A.; Aguiar, A.F.; Léonard, G.; Alves, B.M.O.; Amorim, C.F.; da Silva, R.A. Lumbar stabilisation exercises versus back endurance-resistance exercise training in athletes with chronic low back pain: Protocol of a randomised controlled trial. *BMJ Open Sport Exerc. Med.* **2018**, *4*, e000452. [CrossRef]
17. Bento, T.P.F.; dos Santos Genebra, C.V.; Maciel, N.M.; Cornelio, G.P.; Simeão, S.F.A.P.; de Vitta, A. Low back pain and some associated factors: Is there any difference between genders? *Braz. J. Phys. Ther.* **2020**, *24*, 79–87. [CrossRef]
18. Wu, A.; March, L.; Zheng, X.; Huang, J.; Wang, X.; Zhao, J.; Blyth, F.M.; Smith, E.; Buchbinder, R.; Hoy, D. Global low back pain prevalence and years lived with disability from 1990 to 2017: Estimates from the Global Burden of Disease Study 2017. *Ann. Transl. Med.* **2020**, *8*, 299. [CrossRef]

19. Palacios-Ceña, D.; Albaladejo-Vicente, R.; Hernández-Barrera, V.; Lima-Florencio, L.; Fernández-de-Las-Peñas, C.; Jimenez-Garcia, R.; López-de-Andrés, A.; de Miguel-Diez, J.; Perez-Farinos, N. Female gender is associated with a higher prevalence of chronic neck pain, chronic low back pain, and migraine: Results of the Spanish National Health Survey, 2017. *Pain. Med.* **2021**, *22*, 382–395. [CrossRef]
20. Patil, S.; Mahajan, A. Effect of Graded Plank Protocol on Core Stability in Sedentary Dentists. *Int. J. Res. Rev.* **2020**, *7*, 407–411.
21. Narouei, S.; hossein Barati, A.; Akuzawa, H.; Talebian, S.; Ghiasi, F.; Akbari, A.; hossein Alizadeh, M. Effects of core stabilization exercises on thickness and activity of trunk and hip muscles in subjects with nonspecific chronic low back pain. *J. Bodyw. Mov. Ther.* **2020**, *24*, 138–146. [CrossRef] [PubMed]
22. Kim, S.G.; Yong, M.S.; Na, S.S. The Effect of Trunk Stabilization Exercises with a Swiss Ball on Core Muscle Activation in the Elderly. *J. Phys. Ther. Sci.* **2014**, *26*, 1473–1474. [CrossRef]
23. Akuthota, V.; Ferreiro, A.; Moore, T.; Fredericson, M. Core Stability Exercise Principles. *Curr. Sports Med. Rep.* **2008**, *7*, 39–44. [CrossRef] [PubMed]
24. Miguel, A.; Pardos-Sevilla, A.I.; Jiménez-Fuente, A.; Hubler-Figueiró, T.; d'Orsi, E.; Rech, C.R. Associations of Mutually Exclusive Categories of Physical Activity and Sedentary Time With Metabolic Syndrome in Older Adults: An Isotemporal substitution approach. *J. Aging Phys. Act.* **2021**, *1*, 1–9. [CrossRef]
25. Hopstock, L.A.; Deraas, T.S.; Henriksen, A.; Martiny-Huenger, T.; Grimsgaard, S. Changes in adiposity, physical activity, cardiometabolic risk factors, diet, physical capacity and well-being in inactive women and men aged 57–74 years with obesity and cardiovascular risk–A 6-month complex lifestyle intervention with 6-month follow-up. *PLoS ONE* **2021**, *16*, e0256631. [CrossRef] [PubMed]
26. Lind, L.; Zethelius, B.; Lindberg, E.; Pedersen, N.L.; Byberg, L. Changes in leisure-time physical activity during the adult life span and relations to cardiovascular risk factors—Results from multiple Swedish studies. *PLoS ONE* **2021**, *16*, e0256476. [CrossRef] [PubMed]
27. Park, S.; Nam, J.Y. The Impact of Sedentary Behavior and Self-Rated Health on Cardiovascular Disease and Cancer among South Korean Elderly Persons Using the Korea National Health and Nutrition Examination Survey (KNHANES) 2014–2018 Data. *Int. J. Environ. Res. Public Health* **2021**, *18*, 7426. [CrossRef]
28. García-Unanue, J.; Felipe, J.L.; Bishop, D.; Colino, E.; Ubago-Guisado, E.; López-Fernández, J.; Hernando, E.; Gallardo, L.; Sánchez-Sánchez, J. Muscular and Physical Response to an Agility and Repeated Sprint Tests According to the Level of Competition in Futsal Players. *Front. Psychol.* **2020**, *11*, 3671. [CrossRef]
29. Kim, S.; Jee, Y. Effects of 3D Moving Platform Exercise on Physiological Parameters and Pain in Patients with Chronic Low Back Pain. *Medicina* **2020**, *56*, 351. [CrossRef]
30. Sipaviciene, S.; Kliziene, I.; Pozeriene, J.; Zaicenkoviene, K. Effects of a Twelve-Week Program of Lumbar-Stabilization Exercises on Multifidus Muscles, Isokinetic Peak Torque and Pain for Women with Chronic Low Back Pain. *J. Pain Relief.* **2018**, *7*, 1–10. [CrossRef]
31. Domaszewski, P.; Pakosz, P.; Konieczny, M.; Bączkowicz, D.; Sadowska-Krępa, E. Caffeine-Induced Effects on Human Skeletal Muscle Contraction Time and Maximal Displacement Measured by Tensiomyography. *Nutrients* **2021**, *13*, 815. [CrossRef] [PubMed]
32. Thabet, A.A.; Alshehri, M.A. Efficacy of deep core stability exercise program in postpartum women with diastasis recti abdominis: A randomised controlled trial. *J. Musculoskelet Neuronal. Interact.* **2019**, *19*, 62–68. [PubMed]
33. Križaj, D.; Šimunič, B.; Žagar, T. Short-term repeatability of parameters extracted from radial displacement of muscle belly. *J. Electromyogr. Kinesiol.* **2008**, *18*, 645–651. [CrossRef] [PubMed]
34. Martín-Rodríguez, S.; Loturco, I.; Hunter, A.M.; Rodríguez-Ruiz, D.; Munguia-Izquierdo, D. Reliability and measurement error of tensiomyography to assess mechanical muscle function: A systematic review. *J. Strength Cond. Res.* **2017**, *31*, 3524–3536. [CrossRef] [PubMed]
35. Loturco, I.; Pereira, L.A.; Kobal, R.; Kitamura, K.; Ramírez-Campillo, R.; Zanetti, V.; Abad, C.C.C.; Nakamura, F.Y. Muscle Contraction Velocity: A Suitable Approach to Analyze the Functional Adaptations in Elite Soccer Players. *J. Sports Sci. Med.* **2016**, *15*, 483–491.
36. Lohr, C.; Braumann, K.-M.; Reer, R.; Schroeder, J.; Schmidt, T. Reliability of tensiomyography and myotonometry in detecting mechanical and contractile characteristics of the lumbar erector spinae in healthy volunteers. *Eur. J. Appl. Physiol.* **2018**, *118*, 1349–1359. [CrossRef]
37. Dahmane, R.; Valenčič, V.; Knez, N.; Eržen, I. Evaluation of the ability to make non-invasive estimation of muscle contractile properties on the basis of the muscle belly response. *Med. Biol. Eng. Comput.* **2001**, *39*, 51–55. [CrossRef]
38. Valenčič, V.; Knez, N. Measuring of Skeletal Muscles' Dynamic Properties. *Artif. Organs* **1997**, *21*, 240–242. [CrossRef]
39. Agten, A.; Stevens, S.; Verbrugghe, J.; Eijnde, B.O.; Timmermans, A.; Vandenabeele, F. The lumbar multifidus is characterised by larger type I muscle fibres compared to the erector spinae. *Anat. Cell Biol.* **2020**, *53*, 143–150. [CrossRef]
40. Mannion, A.F.; Dumas, G.A.; Cooper, R.G.; Espinosa, F.; Faris, M.W.; Stevenson, J.M. Muscle fibre size and type distribution in thoracic and lumbar regions of erector spinae in healthy subjects without low back pain: Normal values and sex differences. *J. Anat.* **1997**, *190*, 505–513. [CrossRef]
41. Karp, J.R. Muscle Fiber Types and Training. *Strength Cond. J.* **2001**, *23*, 21–26. [CrossRef]

42. de Paula Simola, R.Á.; Harms, N.; Raeder, C.; Kellmann, M.; Meyer, T.; Pfeiffer, M.; Ferrauti, A. Assessment of Neuromuscular Function After Different Strength Training Protocols Using Tensiomyography. *J. Strength Cond. Res.* **2015**, *29*, 1339–1348. [CrossRef] [PubMed]
43. García-Manso, J.M.; Rodríguez-Matoso, D.; Sarmiento, S.; de Saa, Y.; Vaamonde, D.; Rodríguez-Ruiz, D.; Da Silva-Grigoletto, M.E. Effect of high-load and high-volume resistance exercise on the tensiomyographic twitch response of biceps brachii. *J. Electromyogr. Kinesiol.* **2012**, *22*, 612–619. [CrossRef] [PubMed]
44. García-Manso, J.M.; Rodríguez-Ruiz, D.; Rodríguez-Matoso, D.; de Saa, Y.; Sarmiento, S.; Quiroga, M. Assessment of muscle fatigue after an ultra-endurance triathlon using tensiomyography (TMG). *J. Sports Sci.* **2011**, *29*, 619–625. [CrossRef] [PubMed]
45. Proske, U.; Morgan, D.L. Do cross-bridges contribute to the tension during stretch of passive muscle? *J. Muscle Res. Cell Motil.* **1999**, *20*, 433–442. [CrossRef]
46. Solomonow, M. Neuromuscular manifestations of viscoelastic tissue degradation following high and low risk repetitive lumbar flexion. *J. Electromyogr. Kinesiol.* **2012**, *22*, 155–175. [CrossRef]
47. Wilke, J.; Vogt, L.; Pfarr, T.; Banzer, W. Reliability and validity of a semi-electronic tissue compliance meter to assess muscle stiffness. *J. Back. Musculoskelet Rehabil.* **2018**, *31*, 991–997. [CrossRef]
48. Kenny, G.P.; Reardon, F.D.; Zaleski, W.; Reardon, M.L.; Haman, F.; Ducharme, M.B. Muscle temperature transients before, during, and after exercise measured using an intramuscular multisensor probe. *J. Appl. Physiol.* **2003**, *94*, 2350–2357. [CrossRef]
49. Janecki, D.; Jarocka, E.; Jaskólska, A.; Marusiak, J.; Jaskólski, A. Muscle passive stiffness increases less after the second bout of eccentric exercise compared to the first bout. *J. Sci. Med. Sport* **2011**, *14*, 338–343. [CrossRef]
50. Areeudomwong, P.; Puntumetakul, R.; Jirarattanaphochai, K.; Wanpen, S.; Kanpittaya, J.; Chatchawan, U.; Yamauchi, J. Core Stabilization Exercise Improves Pain Intensity, Functional Disability and Trunk Muscle Activity of Patients with Clinical Lumbar Instability: A Pilot Randomized Controlled Study. *J. Phys. Ther. Sci.* **2012**, *24*, 1007–1012. [CrossRef]
51. Mannion, A.F.; Taimela, S.; Müntener, M.; Dvorak, J. Active Therapy for Chronic Low Back Pain: Part 1. Effects on Back Muscle Activation, Fatigability, and Strength. *Spine* **2001**, *26*, 897–908. [CrossRef] [PubMed]
52. Calatayud, J.; Casaña, J.; Martín, F.; Jakobsen, M.D.; Colado, J.C.; Andersen, L.L. Progression of Core Stability Exercises Based on the Extent of Muscle Activity. *Am. J. Phys. Med. Rehabil.* **2017**, *96*, 694–699. [CrossRef] [PubMed]
53. Ko, K.J.; Kang, S.J. Effects of 12-week core stabilization exercise on the Cobb angle and lumbar muscle strength of adolescents with idiopathic scoliosis. *J. Exerc. Rehabil.* **2017**, *13*, 244–249. [CrossRef] [PubMed]
54. Sekendiz, B.; Cug, M.; Korkusuz, F. Effects of Swiss-ball Core Strength Training on Strength, Endurance, Flexibility, and Balance in Sedentary Women. *J. Strength Cond. Res.* **2010**, *24*, 3032–3040. [CrossRef]
55. Barr, K.P.; Griggs, M.; Cadby, T. Lumbar Stabilization Core Concepts And Current Literature, Part 1. *Am. J. Phys. Med. Rehabil.* **2005**, *84*, 473–480. [CrossRef]
56. Miyake, Y.; Kobayashi, R.; Kelepecz, D.; Nakajima, M. Core exercises elevate trunk stability to facilitate skilled motor behavior of the upper extremities. *J. Bodyw. Mov. Ther.* **2013**, *17*, 259–265. [CrossRef]
57. Granacher, U.; Gollhofer, A.; Hortobágyi, T.; Kressig, R.W.; Muehlbauer, T. The Importance of Trunk Muscle Strength for Balance, Functional Performance, and Fall Prevention in Seniors: A Systematic Review. *Sports Med.* **2013**, *43*, 627–641. [CrossRef]
58. Maeo, S.; Takahashi, T.; Takai, Y.; Kanehisa, H. Trunk Muscle Activities During Abdominal Bracing: Comparison Among Muscles And Exercises. *J. Sports Sci. Med.* **2013**, *12*, 467–474.

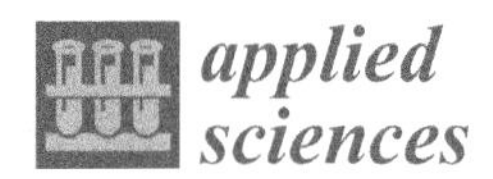

applied sciences

MDPI

Article

The Pattern of Affective Responses to Dance-Based Group Exercise Differs According to Physical Fitness, as Measured by a Smartwatch

Yujin Kim [1], Jihye Kim [2] and Minjung Woo [2,*]

[1] Department of Physical Education, Sejong University, Seoul 05006, Korea; ykim@sju.ac.kr
[2] School of Exercise and Sport Science, University of Ulsan, Ulsan 44610, Korea; rlawlgp1107@naver.com
* Correspondence: mjwoo@ulsan.ac.kr

Abstract: The present study investigated the effect of a dance-based aerobic exercise, on the affective experiences of participants with different fitness levels. Thirty-two college students were enrolled in the same dance fitness course, tested using a physical fitness test (the National Fitness Project 100) and grouped accordingly to 15 sports majors (high-fit group) and 17 non-sports majors (low-fit group). Together, they participated in a single-session dance fitness program using 11 basic dance steps incorporated in Zumba rhythms of merengue and reggaeton for 47 min including warm-up and cool-down. Pre- and post-exercise affects were measured using the PANAS-X transmitted to each participant's smartphone. During exercise, participants' heart rate (HR) and their responses to the felt arousal scale (FAS) and the feeling scale (FS) by exercise section were measured using tailor-made applications on a smartwatch. Results showed that the intensity of exercise for the same exercise program was lower in the high-fit group than in the low-fit group, as evidenced by %HRmax. In addition, the pattern of affective change throughout the exercise sections was different according to the groups' fitness levels, while the affective improvement was greater in the high-fit group. This study confirmed that physical fitness is a major variable influencing the relationship between exercise and affect.

Keywords: affect; physical fitness; dance-based group exercise; wearable technology; smartwatch

Citation: Kim, Y.; Kim, J.; Woo, M. The Pattern of Affective Responses to Dance-Based Group Exercise Differs According to Physical Fitness, as Measured by a Smartwatch. *Appl. Sci.* **2021**, *11*, 11540. https://doi.org/10.3390/app112311540

Academic Editor: Nyeonju Kang

Received: 4 November 2021
Accepted: 2 December 2021
Published: 6 December 2021

1. Introduction

It has been reported that regular exercise has mental health benefits such as reducing depressive symptoms and improving mood and self-esteem [1]. In particular, aerobic exercise is mainly conducive to stress relief and emotional stability, contributing to mental health [2]. In addition, because aerobic exercise has such a powerful effect on depression, some have even referred to it as an antidepressant with no side effects [3].

The psychological benefits of exercise participation vary depending on exercise intensity, duration, and type [4,5]. For example, exercise intensity is a major influencing factor of affect, in that exercise at a moderate to a vigorous intensity below the ventilatory threshold (VT) or lactate threshold (LT) is known to induce positive affective changes [6–9]. One can usually maintain a pleasant affect until the VT, but a sudden shift occurs from a pleasant to unpleasant affect upon exceeding the VT. During exercise at the VT level, the affective experience of individuals gradually declines in the direction of displeasure, which bounces back to pleasure once the exercise completes [6–10]. As such, the affective experience during exercise varies according to the intensity of exercise.

Despite a positive affect restored after exercise, the discomfort experienced during the prior exercise can influence exercise adherence or withdrawal in the future [11]. Therefore, the affective point of view does not recommend immediately exposing beginners to exercise at a high intensity because it is likely to induce negative affective responses during exercise. Furthermore, even with the same exercise program, individuals can feel the intensity of exercise differently depending on their physical fitness level. For example, a moderate-intensity exercise of 60% of HRmax for the high-fit group may be equivalent to a vigorous-intensity exercise of more than 90% of HRmax for the low-physical group [12]. However, little research has investigated how the affective benefit of exercise varies depending on the fitness status of an exerciser.

In a study examining the affective changes during vigorous-intensity exercise in association with exercise intensity preference, the group that preferred low-intensity exercise exhibited gradually increasing displeasure three minutes after the start of the exercise to the end of the exercise (15 min). The affect returned to the pre-exercise level after the exercise. On the other hand, the group that preferred high-intensity exercise maintained the initial level of affect throughout the exercise, and the pleasure increased after the exercise [13]. These results suggest that the impact of exercise on our affective experience can vary significantly according to one's preference for high-intensity exercise. Considering that high-fit individuals have a higher preference for vigorous-intensity exercise than low-fit individuals [14], it can be predicted that there will be differences in affective changes during exercise depending on physical fitness. Therefore, it is of importance to investigate how physical fitness mediates affective experience associated with exercise.

Another important variable that comes into play between exercise and affect is the dynamics experienced when exercising with others. For example, according to the social interaction hypothesis [15] or the psychosocial hypothesis [16], the interaction between people participating in exercise or positive attention from those exercising together is a key factor in affective improvement we receive from exercise. Furthermore, the degree to which exercise increases endorphins is greater when a group is together than alone [17]. A rhythmic exercise accompanied by music may add benefit to the mood-lifting effect [18,19]. In this regard, considering the dynamic factors involved in the effect of exercise on affect, researchers should conduct studies on the exercise–affect relationship in a real-life exercise field rather than in a laboratory setting.

To date, the existing research tools have not been capable of accurately measuring the constantly changing affect and exercise intensity (heart rates) at the same time, particularly for a large group of people in the exercise field. However, with the recent development of the Internet of things (IoT), several wearable devices have been introduced [20]. Of these devices, the smartwatch enables us to send, respond, and collect questionnaires and measure the heart rate required for identifying exercise intensity and automatically store all the data in the cloud. Smartwatches generally use photoplethysmographic (PPG) signals to measure heart rate [21]. Prior studies verified the accuracy and reliability of heart rate measured with smartwatches in varying conditions (e.g., rest, walking, cycling, dancing) [22]. In addition, it is possible to control multiple smartwatches simultaneously, transmit and store data automatically via an application developed to suit the purpose. Thus, wearable devices and mobile apps have made field research possible beyond existing research tools.

Zumba fitness is one of the representative dance-based sports that have recently dominated the group exercise market. Zumba fitness is a workout program that blends energetic Latin music with basic dance steps in a fitness program that encourages participants to enjoy aerobic exercise and have fun, as indicated by its official motto, "Ditch the workout. Join the party" [23]. The exercise intensity of Zumba is known to be 66 $\pm$ 10.5% of the average VO2max, consuming 369 $\pm$ 108 Kcal for 40 min [24], which meets the American College of Sports Medicine (ACSM)'s recommended dose to maintain a healthy weight [25]. Research evidence suggests that Zumba effectively improves aerobic fitness [26] and weight loss [27]. In addition, participation in Zumba fitness enhances positive affect. In a recent study, Lee et al. [28] investigated the affective changes during Zumba fitness as a function of exercise intensity. They found that 45-min low-intensity and moderate-intensity Zumba programs both affected improving effect during exercise, with greater positive affect observed in moderate intensity relative to low intensity. Furthermore, Zumba fitness improves quality of life [29] and alleviate depressive symptoms [30].

Therefore, this study uses a smartwatch in a real-life exercise setting to investigate the effect of a dance-based aerobic group class on the affective experiences of participants with different fitness levels.

2. Materials and Methods

2.1. Participants

Thirty-two sports major (n = 15, 23.33 ± 1.88 years old) and non-major (n = 17, 20.59 ± 1.67 years old) college students were enrolled in the same dance fitness course and voluntarily participated in the present study. A physical fitness test was conducted on each participant. Based on these results, the participants were classified according to physical fitness into high-fit and low-fit groups (Table 1). Participants were instructed to refrain from alcohol intake 24 h before the experiment and excessive exercise 72 h before the experiment. The authors' Institutional Review Board (1040968-A-2020-020) approved the research protocol for this study. The sample size required for this research design was estimated using the G*power calculator (version 3.1.9.4; Düsseldorf University, Düsseldorf, Germany) [31]. The sample size was estimated based on a significance level of 0.05, the statistical power of 0.90, and the effect size found in a previous study investigating affective changes during a group dance program (η^2 = 0.497). Based on these criteria, the estimated sample size was 18 people, meaning that nine or more participants in each high-fit and low-fit group would yield a statistical power above 0.90. Therefore, the number of participants in this study (n = 32) is expected to have sufficient statistical power.

Table 1. Demographic information of participants.

Item	High-Fit Group		Low-Fit Group	
	M	*SD*	*M*	*SD*
Age (yrs.)	23.33	1.88	20.59	1.67
BMI (kg/m^2)	23.56	3.96	22.63	3.84
Body fat (%)	25.09	6.94	31.87	7.94
Fitness (Z-score)	0.36	0.69	−0.52	0.56

2.2. Materials

2.2.1. Physical Fitness Measures

To measure the participants' physical fitness, the National Fitness Project 100 developed by the Korean Ministry of Culture, Sports and Tourism was used [32,33]. This measure consists of six categories: muscular strength (grip strength), muscular endurance (cross sit-ups), cardiorespiratory endurance (20 m shuttle run), flexibility (seated forward bend), agility (4 × 10 m shuttle run), and power (standing long jump). The fitness outcome values for all six categories were standardized into Z scores to minimize the influence of age and gender variables using the mean and standard deviation of the population (men and women in the early 20 s) provided by the Ministry of Culture, Sports and Tourism [33] (Formula (1)).

$$Z\ score_{ij} = \frac{Y_{ij} - \overline{Y_i}}{S_Y} \quad (1)$$

(i: participants, j: fitness category, Y: fitness score, $\overline{Y}$: population mean, S_Y: population SD).

After obtaining the total fitness scores by averaging the standardized Z scores in all fitness categories for individual participants, an independent sample t-test was performed to verify the difference in the physical fitness measure between the groups. Results showed that the overall fitness score of the high-fit group (Z = 0.36) was higher than that of the low-fit group (Z = −0.52) (t = 3.96, p < 0.001) (Table 1).

2.2.2. Smartphone

An android-based smartphone (Galaxy Note 9, Samsung, Seoul, Korea) was used where we installed a tailor-made app for remote control of the smartwatches and monitoring the measurement status. For data collection on arousal and affective responses of participants during Zumba fitness, all the smartwatches worn by the participants were controlled simultaneously by this single central smartphone.

2.2.3. Smartwatch

TicWatch E (Mobvoi, Beijing, China) was used, an Android Wear OS 2.0-based smartwatch capable of running our tailor-made app and equipped with a GPS, heart rate (HR) sensor, proximity sensor, balance sensor, and accelerometer. TicWatch E has reliable accuracy, showing more than 95% correlation and agreement than the HR measured by Polar (wireless HR monitor, POLAR) during walking, dancing, and cycling as well as at rest [22]. Because the smartwatch's adhesion to the wearer's skin can impair HR measurement accuracy [34]. Kinesiology tape was applied around the watch to reduce movement and loss of light from the sensor during workouts. The watch was securely fastened to the participant's left wrist, approximately 2–3 cm below the ulnar styloid process. All participants wore smartwatches, measuring heart rate, arousal, and mood during Zumba fitness exercise.

2.2.4. Application Development and Smartwatch Control

In collaboration with a software engineering expert, an application was developed to collect HR and affective data and another one to control smartwatches. The app installed on the smartphone for the measurement of HR and affect was to activate the HR sensor of smartwatch to initiate HR measurement and to collect data via participants' affective self-reports, which was designed to be stored automatically on Google Cloud. A watch control app was also developed on the Galaxy S9 with Android Pie (version 9.0) to ensure that the measurement app operated effectively on the smartwatch. The watch control app comprised four modes: watch connection, HR measurement, affect measurement, and data management. In the "watch connection" mode, the connection status of up to 30 smartwatches was monitored. The "HR measurement" mode was used to initialize, start, pause, or stop the smartwatch HR sensor. In the "affect measurement" mode, a vibration alarm was sent to the participants on their smartwatches, which cued to report current feelings and arousal states by selecting responses on the watch's touch screen. The HR and affective data were stored in the Google Cloud for real time monitoring (Figure 1). All data acquired during the experiment were freely accessible to be downloaded or deleted via the "data management mode".

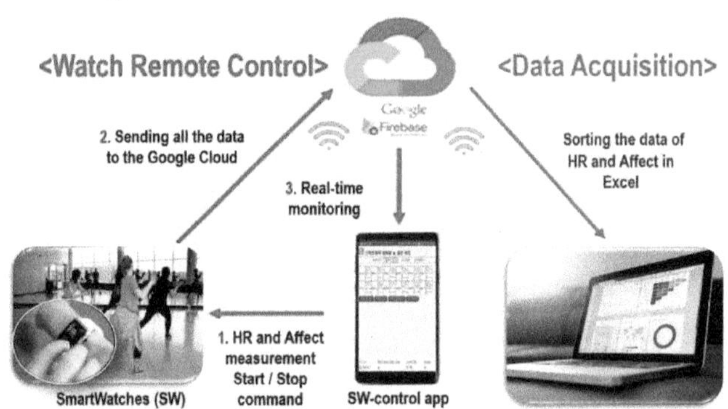

Figure 1. Description of smartwatch control and data acquisition processes.

2.3. *Affective Measures*

2.3.1. Positive and Negative Affect Schedule-Expanded Form (PANAS-X)

To measure the affective changes before and after Zumba fitness, the Korean version of the Positive Affect and Negative Affect Schedule—expanded form (PANAS-X) was used [35]. The PANAS-X is a five-point 20-item scale comprising 10 positive and 10 negative items (i.e., 1 = not at all, 2 = a little, 3 = moderately, 4 = quite a bit, 5 = very much).

With an internal consistency coefficient of 0.84, the PANAS-X scale is relatively reliable, and the positive and negative affect scales are independent. We created the online version of the 20-item PANAS-X with Google Forms and transmitted the link to the smartphones of study participants for a response. Their responses were stored automatically on Google Drive. In the present study, the Cronbach's alpha coefficients were 0.61 for the PA and 0.66 for the NA scales.

2.3.2. Two-Dimensional Circumplex Model of Affect

Russell 's [36] two-dimensional circumplex was used to track the affective changes throughout the entire Zumba Fitness program. As presented in Figure 2, the model consists of four quadrants, each of which represents arousal level (activation–deactivation continuum) and valence (pleasure–displeasure continuum). In the two-dimensional circumplex model, the affective state can be identified by the point of intersection, with the x and y axes signifying valence (pleasure, displeasure) and arousal (activation–deactivation continuum), respectively (Figure 2). Russell [37] defined this intersecting point as a core affect reflecting valence and activation. The valence dimension was assessed by the feeling scale (FS), while the arousal dimension reflected the felt arousal scale (FAS).

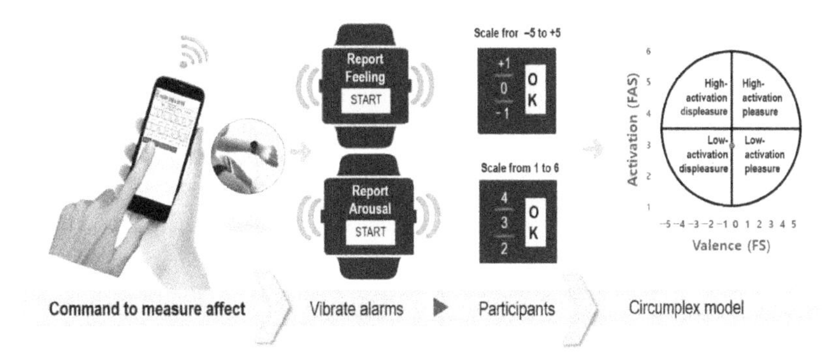

Figure 2. The two-dimensional circumplex model of affect and the smartwatch display for measuring affect and arousal.

This model consists of four quadrants: The first quadrant describes activation–pleasure (excited, energized, and passionate), while the second quadrant reflects activation–displeasure (anxious, nervous, and stressed). The third quadrant represents deactivation–displeasure (bored, tired, and depressed), and the fourth quadrant represents deactivation–pleasure (relaxed and calm) [36]. The smartwatch interface was used to implement the feeling scale (FS) and the felt arousal scale (FAS) to simultaneously evaluate affect in multiple participants engaging in the group exercise concurrently.

2.3.3. The Feeling Scale (FS)

A single item 11-point bipolar FS (pleasure/displeasure) devised by Hardy and Rejeski [38] was used to assess during exercise affective responses on the valence dimension (x-axis) of the two-dimensional circumplex model of affect. When participants received a vibration alarm sent from the central watch control app with the message "report Feeling" on the smartwatch screen, the app guided participants to press the start button and scroll up or down the touch screen to choose a number from −5 to +5 corresponding to their current feelings (Figure 2). The Cronbach's alpha coefficient of the FS in the present study was 0.89.

2.3.4. The Felt Arousal Scale (FAS)

The FAS devised by Svebak and Murgatroyd [39] was used to evaluate the level of arousal on the arousal dimension (y-axis) of the two-dimensional circumplex model. This single-item six-point scale ranging from 1 (low arousal or deactivation) to 6 (high arousal or activation) was used to assess arousal levels during exercise. When the "report arousal" screen appeared on participants' smartwatches with a vibration alarm, the participants chose a number from 1 to 6 corresponding to their current activation status. Then, they sent the response by pressing the OK button (Figure 2). The Cronbach's alpha coefficient of the FAS in the present study was 0.73.

2.4. Dance Fitness Program

The dance fitness program was developed using 11 basic dance steps incorporated in Zumba rhythms of merengue and reggaeton, consisting of 8-min warp-up, 8-min basic steps, 8-min merengue, 8-min reggaeton, 15-min cool-down with stretching, all totaling 47-min of exercise. Table 2 presents the details of the steps, music, and beat per minute used in the program.

Table 2. Dance fitness program.

Rhythm	Basic Steps				Music	bpm
Aerobics	March, step touch, V-step, lunge, heel-jack, knee up, grapevine, mambo, back-up, box, tap				Top Ten 24 #1	130
Merengue	March	2 Step	6 Step	Beto Shuffle	Basic 1 review music Fiesta	124 124
Reggaeton	Stomp	Knee-lift	Destroza	Step bounce	Basic 1 review music Toma reggaeton	94 96

2.5. Procedures

Participants who signed the informed consent visited the National Fitness 100 Center to have their physical fitness measured, required for completion 72 h before the experiment. When participants arrived, the smartwatch firmly fitted on their left wrist, 2 to 3 cm below the ulnar styloid process. Then, they were instructed to sit and rest on a yoga mat. The experimenter then initiated the watch control app on the smartphone, checked the connection of all watches, and tested if the alarm transmission and HR measurement worked properly. After explaining the experimental procedure, we transmitted the 20-item PANAS-X to each participant's smartphone to be answered before beginning the exercise. To begin the Zumba fitness program, participants stood with enough space between them and faced the mirror. At the start of the session, the experimenter activated the HR sensors of participants' smartwatches by pressing the start button of the HR measurement mode of the watch control app. At the end of each exercise section (warm-up, basic steps, merengue, reggaeton), the experimenter hit the stop button of the watch control app to finish HR measurement and transmitted an alarm in the affect measurement mode. Once all the participants completed responding to the FS and FAS scales by touching the smartwatch screen, the watch control app confirmed the completed responses, and the group proceeded to the next exercise section.

As shown in Figure 3, the PANAS-X pre-and post-exercise and the HR during exercise (warm-up, basic steps, merengue, reggaeton) were measured. The FS and FAS were measured six times (pre-exercise after PANAS-X, 8 min, 17 min, 26 min, 35 min, and post-exercise before PANAS-X). The time required for answering the FS and FAS in between sections was 20 to 40 s. When the Zumba program was over with reggaeton, followed by a cool-down, participants responded to the post-exercise FS and FAS while resting on the yoga mat. Then, the PANAS-X link was sent to the participants' smartphones to respond. After completing the response and returning the watch to the experimenter, participants returned home.

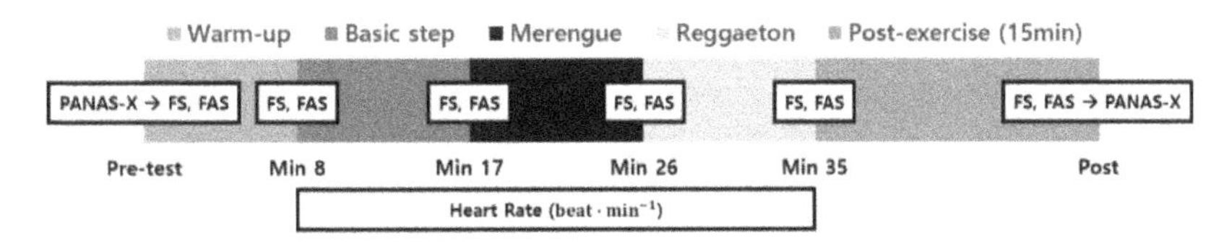

Figure 3. The measurement of HR, affect, and arousal before, during, and after exercise.

2.6. Data Collection and Processing

The HR measured during exercise by section (warm-up: exercise start to 8 min, basic step: 8–17 min, merengue: 17–26 min, reggaeton: 26 min to completion) were averaged to verify whether a difference existed in the exercise intensity of the dance exercise program between the high-fit and low-fit groups. Then, the relative exercise intensity of the participants was calculated using the HR data and the HRmax estimation formula (HRmax = 220-age) [25,40]. Finally, the exercise intensity was calculated by dividing the HRmax by the during-exercise HR, multiplied by 100 [41].

2.7. Statistical Analysis

All statistical analyses were performed using the SPSS Version 25.0 for Windows. Mauchly's sphericity test was performed on all dependent variables and adjusted the degree of freedom of ANOVA through Greenhouse–Geisser for variables that did not meet the sphericity assumption. The level of statistical significance of ANOVAs was set to 0.05, and the significance level for HR and exercise intensity was 0.0031 for post-hoc analysis. The significance levels for the PANAS-X and the FS and FAS were 0.0125 and 0.0014, respectively. An analysis of variance (ANOVA) was performed to investigate the interaction of HR, exercise intensity, PANAS-X, FS, and FAS as a function of group and time. To examine differences in HR and exercise intensity, separate 2 (group: high-fit vs. low-fit) × 4 (time: warm-up, basic steps, merengue, reggaeton) two-way repeated-measures ANOVAs were performed. In addition, the positive and negative affect of the PANAS-X was analyzed by a 2 (group: high-fit vs. low-fit) × 2 (time: pre- vs. post-exercise) two-way repeated-measures ANOVA. Finally, separate 2 (group: high-fit vs. low-fit) × 6 (time: pre-exercise, 8 min, 17 min, 26 min, 35 min, post-exercise) two-way repeated-measures ANOVAs were performed using FS and FAS as dependent variables. In case of an interaction effect between the group and time, a post-hoc analysis was performed. The significance level was set through Bonferroni adjustment for all post-hoc analyses.

3. Results

3.1. HR and Exercise Intensity (%HRmax)

In the analysis of HR by measurement time, significant group ($F(1, 30) = 20.646$, $p < 0.001$, $d = 1.18$, CI [0.79, 2.40]) and time ($F(2.2, 30) = 12.936$, $p < 0.001$, $d = 1.66$, CI[0.88, 1.77]) main effects emerged. The HR of the high-fit group during exercise was lower than that of the low-fit group ($p < 0.001$) (Figure 4).

As a result of post-hoc analysis of the main effect of time, the HR during basic steps ($p = 0.002$) and reggaeton exercise ($p < 0.001$) was higher than the HR during the warm-up exercise, and the HR during reggaeton exercise was higher than the HR during the merengue exercise ($p < 0.001$). In the analysis of exercise intensity, calculated by %HRmax, significant main effects of group ($F(1, 30) = 17.522$, $p < 0.001$, $d = 1.53$, CI[1 0.05, 2.09]) and time ($F(2.197, 30) = 12.882$, $p < 0.001$, $d = 1.31$, CI[0.88, 1.76]) emerged, with the high-fit group exhibiting lower exercise intensity compared to the low-fit group ($p < 0.001$). The post-hoc analysis on the main effect of time revealed that the exercise intensity of the basic steps ($p = 0.002$) and reggaeton exercise ($p < 0.001$) was higher than that of the warm-up exercise, and the exercise intensity of reggaeton was higher than that of merengue ($p < 0.001$). However, the interaction for group × time was not significant in HR and exercise intensity.

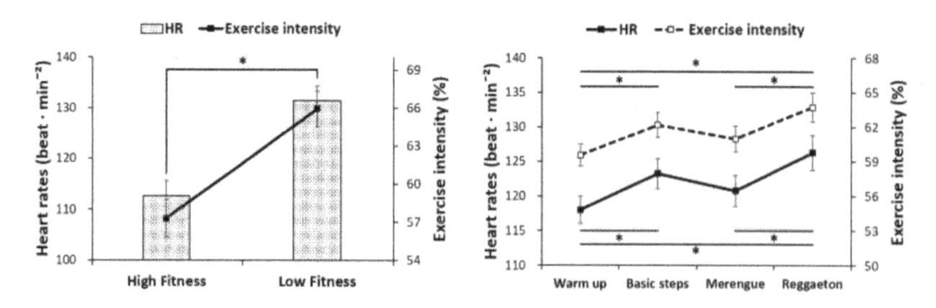

Figure 4. Differences in heart rates and the exercise intensity between groups (**left**) and times (**right**). Note: all the error bars represent standard errors. In the difference between times (**left**), the significant value adjusted by Bonferroni correlation is $p < 0.0031$. * represents a significant difference.

3.2. PANAS-X

3.2.1. Positive Affect

A significant main effect of group emerged ($F(1, 30) = 5.585$, $p = 0.025$, $d = 0.86$, CI[0.59, 1.18]), with the high-fit group exhibiting higher positive affect relative to the low-fit group. However, the main effect on time was not significant. As a result of ANOVA before and after exercise between groups, we found a significant interaction effect between groups × period ($F(1, 30) = 8.261$, $p = 0.007$, $d = 1.05$, CI[0.72, 1.44]). The post-hoc analysis revealed no significant group difference in pre-exercise positive affect. Meanwhile, the post-exercise positive affect was significantly higher in the high-fit group compared to the low-fit group ($p = 0.003$) (Figure 5). However, no significant difference was observed in positive affect between pre- and post-exercise within each group.

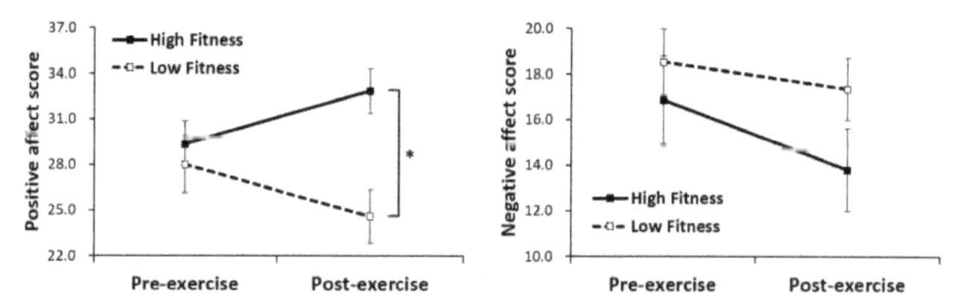

Figure 5. Differences in positive (**left**) and negative (**right**) affective responses between groups and times. Note: solid lines represent the high fitness group, and dash lines represent the low fitness group. All error bars speak of standard errors. $p < 0.0125$. * represents a significant difference.

3.2.2. Negative Affect

The analysis of pre- and post-exercise negative affect between groups yielded no significant main effect or interaction effect (Figure 5).

3.3. The Feeling Scale and Felt Arousal Scale

3.3.1. The Feeling Scale

In the analysis of the FS, there was a significant main effect of time on the FS scores ($F(3.3, 30) = 14.306$, $p < 0.001$, $d = 1.38$, CI[0.91, 1.83]), while the main effect of group did not reach significance. In addition, a significant group × time interaction effect ($F(3.3, 30) = 3.192$, $p = 0.023$, $d = 0.65$, CI[0.43, 0.86]) emerged (Figure 6). As a result of the post-hoc analysis, the high-fit group showed significantly higher FS scores at 26 min and 35 min than pre-exercise ($p < 0.001389$). In contrast, the low-fit group exhibited higher FS scores after exercise than pre-exercise, 17 min, 26 min, and 35 min ($p < 0.001389$). However, no significant difference emerged between the groups as a function of time.

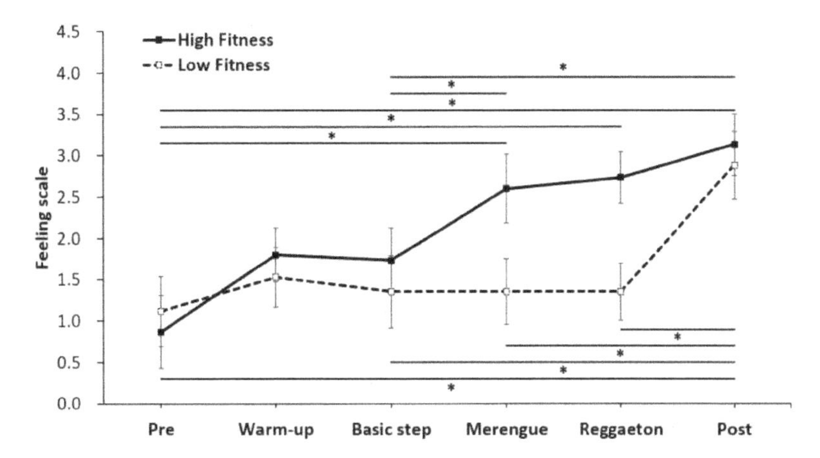

Figure 6. Differences in the feeling scale between groups and times. Note: solid lines represent the high fitness group, and the dashed line represents the low fitness group. All error bars speak of standard errors. $p < 0.0014$. * represents a significant difference.

3.3.2. The Felt Arousal Scale

In the analysis of the FAS scores, a significant main effect of time emerged ($F(3.3, 30) = 9.916$, $p < 0.001$, $d = 1.15$, CI[0.76, 1.52]), but the main effect of group was not significant. A group × time interaction effect was also significant ($F(3.1, 30) = 2.968$, $p = 0.034$, $d = 0.63$, CI[0.42, 0.83]) (Figure 7). The post hoc analysis revealed that the FAS score of the high-fit group was higher at 26 min compared to pre-exercise, 8 min, and 17 min, and the score was also higher at 35 min compared to pre-exercise and 17 min ($p < 0.001389$). However, the low-fit group exhibited no significant difference in the FAS score depending on time, with no group × time interaction.

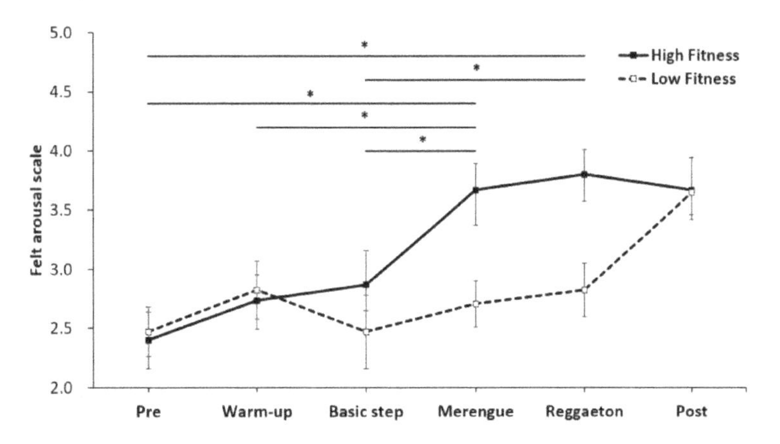

Figure 7. Differences in the felt arousal scale between groups and times. Note: solid lines represent the high fitness group, and the dashed line represents the low fitness group. All error bars speak of standard errors, $p < 0.0014$. * represents a significant difference.

3.4. The Two-Dimensional Circumplex Model

According to time by group, the affective changes are depicted in a two-dimensional circumplex model of valence and activation in Figure 8. For example, the core affect of the low-fit group remained in the fourth quadrant (deactivation–pleasure) without significant change from pre-exercise at 35 min. It then moved to the first quadrant (activation–pleasure) after exercise. On the other hand, the core affect of the high-fit group gradually improved within the fourth quadrant (deactivation–pleasure) from pre-exercise. Finally, it advanced to the first quadrant (activation–pleasure) after 26 min (merengue), which participants maintained until exercise completion.

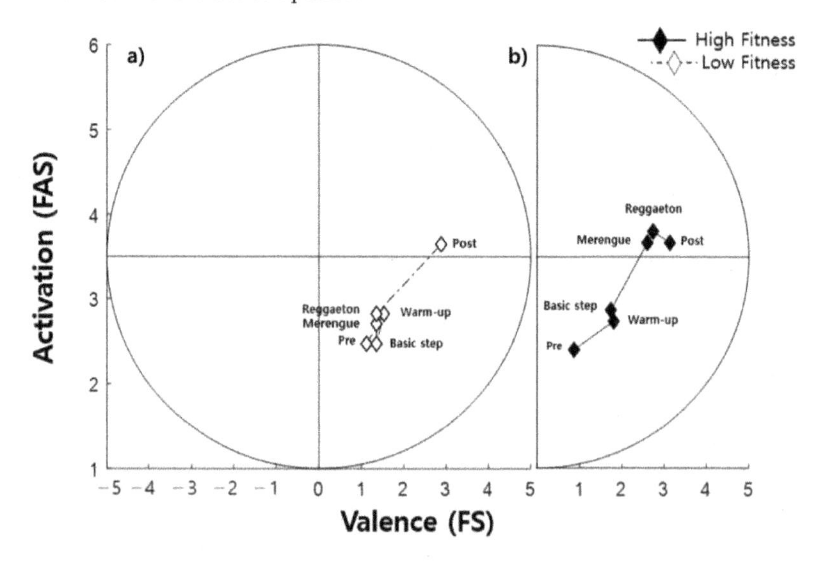

Figure 8. Two-dimensional circumplex model of affect by the level of fitness, (**a**) high fitness and (**b**) low fitness. Note: the circumplex model is a method to observe a change of 'core' affect (valence + activation). Quadrant I represents activation–pleasure; Quadrant II represents activation–displeasure; Quadrant III represents deactivation–displeasure; Quadrant IV represents deactivation–pleasure.

4. Discussion

This study used a smartwatch to investigate whether a dance-based aerobic group exercise affects participants' affective responses depending on their level of physical fitness. In the analysis of the difference in exercise intensity of Zumba fitness according to physical fitness, the high-fit and low-fit groups exhibited differences in HR and exercise intensity (%HRmax) during 35 min of Zumba exercise from warm-up to just before cool-down. Specifically, HR during exercise was 109 bpm with 57% HRmax exercise intensity for the high-fit group and 130 bpm with 66% HRmax intensity for the low-fit group.

The ACSM [25] indicated that the relative intensity of aerobic exercise is 57–63% HRmax for low intensity and 64–76% HRmax for moderate intensity. Therefore, the Zumba fitness program used in this study is of moderate intensity for the low-fit individuals and low-intensity for the high-fit participants. This study's Zumba exercise intensity supports the findings of Luettgen et al. [24] that the exercise intensity of Zumba for the general public is 66 $\pm$ 10.5% of the average VO2max, which meets the ACSM criteria for maintaining a healthy weight. Furthermore, by tracking HR during exercise in real-time using a smartwatch, our study verified that exercise intensity differs depending on the performer's fitness level. Our study's Zumba fitness program consisted of a warm-up, basic dance steps, merengue, and reggaeton. In the comparison of exercise intensity according to the exercise section, we found that the exercise intensity of reggaeton was the highest compared to warm-up, basic steps, and merengue. This result is consistent with Lee et al. [28], who reported the highest HR during reggaeton exercise among the four Zumba rhythms: merengue, reggaeton, salsa, and cumbia. While merengue consists of up-down movements of the pelvis, reggaeton creates up-down motions of the entire lower body through flexion and extension, thus intensifying the exercise. In addition, since the reggaeton steps use two steps per 1 bpm [42], it is possible to double up the speed of the movements up to 192 bpm [43]. Therefore, to control the intensity of a Zumba fitness program within a limited time, instructors often control the speed of choreography by adding or subtracting the portion of reggaeton rhythm or breaking down the rhythm.

In the analysis of the change in affect (valence) and arousal (activation) by exercise section of the Zumba fitness program, we found an interesting difference between the high-fit and low-fit groups. There was no significant change in high-fit group's affect from pre-exercise, warm-up, and basic steps. However, the affect improved after the merengue, and participants maintained that affect throughout the rest of the exercise program. On the other hand, there were no significant changes in affect throughout the entire exercise section in the low-fit group, but the affect improved immediately after the cool-down. Furthermore, similar affective changes were observed in pre, mid, and post-exercise depending on fitness in arousal. In the high-fit group, arousal increased after merengue, and participants maintained this affect until the end. In contrast, the low-fit group showed no difference between pre and during-exercise arousal.

As shown in the two-dimensional circumplex model, which presents the changes in the core affect (valence + activation) (Figure 8), the core affect of the high-fit group increased from the beginning. It proceeded to the first quadrant after merengue, and the participants maintained the affect until the end of the exercise. The low-fit group maintained the core affect without significant change in the fourth quadrant, including their pre-exercise state and throughout the entire section. They then moved to the first quadrant immediately after exercise, showing increased positive affect and arousal. These findings suggest that despite the shared feelings of elevated mood and arousal individuals feel after exercise, the affective experience during exercise may differ depending on participants' fitness level. In addition, high-fit individuals seem to experience a greater increase in affect throughout the exercise than low-fit individuals.

For quick and repeated measurement of changes in affect and arousal in real-time during exercise, a single item 11-point Likert scale (−5 to +5) was used. In doing so, we only assessed the affective experience during exercise within the extent of high and low levels of valence (displeasure to pleasure) and arousal (deactivation to activation). To supplement this, the participants were asked to answer a 20-item PANAS-X to measure positive and negative affect before and after exercise. The results of the PANAS-X pre- and post-exercise and the results of affect (valence) measured by the FS pre-, during-, and post-exercise were not consistent. Figure 5 shows that the high-fit and low-fit groups did not differ in positive affect before exercise. However, the positive affect after exercise was higher in the high-fit group relative to the low-fit group.

Despite no statistical difference between groups as a function of time (pre and post-exercise), positive affect increased after exercise in the high-fit group and decreased in the low-fit group. This tendency made the difference in positive affect between groups significant after exercise. However, we found no significant difference in negative affect according to the fitness level or time in this study, which suggests that participation in a group dance program such as Zumba fitness may not lead to meaningful changes in negative affect. These results are consistent with the study of Lee et al. [28], where negative affect measured before and after a Zumba fitness program was not different regardless of exercise intensity. This finding implies that improved positive affect rather than decreased negative affect provides the affective benefit in dance-based exercise.

Interestingly, the results of this study regarding pre and post-exercise affect are somewhat contradictory to previous studies that investigated affective changes following exercise. The existing studies primarily focused on exploring affective changes according to exercise intensity. Many of them reported that moderate-intensity exercise could expect a greater affective improvement than exercises at a too low or high intensity [44]. In a recent study by Lee et al. [28] which investigated affective changes before, during, and after exercise of Zumba fitness depending on exercise intensity, moderate-intensity (72.19% HRmax) exercise led to a greater increase in positive affect than low-intensity (62.48% HRmax) exercise. Lee et al. also found that affect and arousal during exercise at moderate intensity gradually increased. In contrast, low-intensity exercise only led to a temporary increase in positive affect at the beginning of the exercise, without additional improvement during and after the exercise. Therefore, the researchers suggested that the affective benefit of exercise is greater when performed at moderate intensity than at low intensity. Our results contradict previous studies: we found that low-intensity (i.e., 57% HRmax in high-fit group) exercise provides more significant affective benefit than moderate-intensity (i.e., 66% HRmax in low-fit group) exercise. However, the characteristics of the physical fitness variable need to be considered which influence the exercise–affect relationship.

Physical fitness is about moving the body to carry out a healthy and active daily life, which is the foundation of normal life [45]. Regular exercise enhances fitness [11]. Rezazadeh and Talebi [46] investigated how physical fitness mediates affective responses in firefighters and reported a positive correlation between physical fitness and affect and a negative correlation between BMI and affect. They concluded that since high-fit individuals have better emotional regulation ability, improving the fitness of firefighters would contribute to enhancing their work efficiency. Furthermore, individuals with higher aerobic fitness have a higher tolerance for exercise and a preference for high-intensity exercise [14]. The emotional regulation ability and exercise tolerance demonstrated in high-fit individuals are related to neurological and biological changes caused by long-term exercise participation.

In this study, although the high-fit group exercised at a lower intensity than the low-fit group, they exhibited a greater increase in positive affect, with affect and activation increasing faster during exercise and increasing gradually. Lin and Kuo [47] explained the benefits of exercise on brain function through monoamine connection. They indicated that regular moderate-intensity exercise improves adaptability and flexibility of the central nervous system (CNS). Exercise stimulates the monoaminergic systems (dopamine, noradrenaline, serotonin), thereby contributing to mental health without causing central fatigue. In addition, experiencing a repetitive increase in serotonin in the brain through regular exercise is known to act as an antidepressant [48]. Regular exercise participation also improves biological adaptation, which reduces physiological responses to stress [49]. Since exercise itself is a stressor, exposure to repeated exercise improves adaptability to stress and reduces the secretion of cortisol, a stress hormone, during exercise [50]. Having gained the ability to adapt to stress through regular exercise, high-fit individuals exhibit low levels of salivary cortisol secretion even in exercise-irrelevant stress situations [51,52]. As such, the neurophysiological changes due to long-term exercise participation may explain why the high-fit group in this study showed larger affective improvement than the low-fit group.

Physical fitness is a vital variable mediating affective experience during exercise. In this study, the pattern of affective change throughout the exercise sections was different according to the groups' fitness levels. The intensity of exercise for the same exercise program was lower in the high-fit group than in the low-fit group, while the affective improvement was greater in the high-fit group. This study confirmed that physical fitness is a major variable influencing the relationship between exercise and affect. However, we could not establish how fitness mediates affect through interaction with exercise intensity. Therefore, future studies should examine the interaction between fitness and exercise intensity to identify exercise conditions optimized for affective benefit.

In addition, developing a personalized exercise program that induces optimal affective improvement requires investigating the individual variables that mediate affective responses to exercise and the environmental variables that maximize the effect of exercise. In this regard, artificial neural networks or deep learning technology will become the ultimate goal of future exercise–affect research. This technology can aid in developing an algorithm capable of predicting and suggesting the best suitable exercise type, intensity, and duration based on individual (e.g., personality, physical fitness, genes, diseases) and environmental variables (e.g., exercise type, setting, interaction with others during exercise).

Moreover, deep learning technology could maximize the overall mental health benefit of exercise.

Author Contributions: Conceptualization, M.W.; project administration, J.K. and M.W.; data analysis, J.K.; writing—original draft, M.W.; writing—translating and editing, Y.K.; manuscript preparation, Y.K.; supervision, M.W.; funding acquisition, M.W. All authors have read and agreed to the published version of the manuscript.

Funding: This work was supported by the Ministry of Education of the Republic of Korea and the National Research Foundation of Korea (NRF-2020S1A5A2A01045029).

Institutional Review Board Statement: The study was conducted according to the guidelines of the Declaration of Helsinki, and approved by the Institutional Review Board (or Ethics Committee) of University of Ulsan (1040968-A-2020-020).

Informed Consent Statement: Informed consent was obtained from all subjects involved in the study.

Conflicts of Interest: The authors declared no potential conflict of interest with respect to the research, authorship, and/or publication of this article.

References

1. White, K.; Kendrick, T.; Yardley, L. Change in self-esteem, self-efficacy and the mood dimensions of depression as potential mediators of the physical activity and depression relationship: Exploring the temporal relation of change. *Ment. Health Phys. Act.* **2009**, *2*, 44–52. [CrossRef]
2. Dimeo, F.; Bauer, M.; Varahram, I.; Proest, G.; Halter, U. Benefits from aerobic exercise in patients with major depression: A pilot study. *Br. J. Sports Med.* **2001**, *35*, 114–117. [CrossRef] [PubMed]
3. Sigwalt, A.R.; Budde, H.; Helmich, I.; Glaser, V.; Ghisoni, K.; Lanza, S.; Cadore, E.L.; Lhullier, F.L.; de Bem, A.F.; Hohl, A.; et al. Molecular aspects involved in swimming exercise training reducing anhedonia in a rat model of depression. *Neuroscience* **2011**, *192*, 661–674. [CrossRef]
4. Buckworth, J.; Dishman, R. Determinants of exercise and physical activity. In *Exercise Psychology*; Human Kinetics: Champaign, IL, USA, 2002; pp. 191–209.
5. Mun, C. The Effects of Preference Mode and Intensity of Exercise on Participants' Psychological and Physiological Responses. *Korean J. Sport Psychol.* **2011**, *22*, 149–169.
6. Bixby, W.R.; Lochbaum, M.R. Affect Responses to Acute Bouts of Aerobic Exercise in Fit and Unfit Participants: An Examination of Opponent-Process Theory. *J. Sport Behav.* **2006**, *29*, 111–125.
7. Ekkekakis, P.; Hall, E.E.; Petruzzello, S.J. The relationship between exercise intensity and affective responses demystified: To crack the 40-year-old nut, replace the 40-year-old nutcracker! *Ann. Behav. Med.* **2008**, *35*, 136–149. [CrossRef] [PubMed]
8. Kilpatrick, M.; Kraemer, R.; Bartholomew, J.; Acevedo, E.; Jarreau, D. Affective responses to exercise are dependent on intensity rather than total work. *Med. Sci. Sports Exerc.* **2007**, *39*, 1417–1422. [CrossRef]
9. Sheppard, K.E.; Parfitt, G. Acute Affective Responses to Prescribed and Self-Selected Exercise Intensities in Young Adolescent Boys and Girls. *Pediatr. Exerc. Sci.* **2008**, *20*, 129–141. [CrossRef] [PubMed]
10. Rose, E.A.; Parfitt, G. A quantitative analysis and qualitative explanation of the individual differences in affective responses to prescribed and self-selected exercise intensities. *J. Sport Exerc. Psychol.* **2007**, *29*, 281–309. [CrossRef]
11. Williams, D.M.; Rhodes, R.E.; Conner, M.T. (Eds.) Psychological hedonism, hedonic motivation, and health behavior. In *Affective Determinants of Health Behavior*; Oxford University Press: New York, NY, USA, 2018; pp. 204–234.
12. Physical Activity Guidelines Advisory Committee. *Physical Activity Guidelines Advisory Committee Report*; Department of Health and Human Services: Washington, DC, USA, 2008.
13. Box, A.G.; Petruzzello, S.J. Why do they do it? Differences in high-intensity exercise-affect between those with higher and lower intensity preference and tolerance. *Psychol. Sport Exerc.* **2020**, *47*, 101521. [CrossRef]
14. Schneider, M.; Graham, D. Personality, physical fitness, and affective response to exercise among adolescents. *Med. Sci. Sports Exerc.* **2009**, *41*, 947. [CrossRef]
15. Turner, J.H. *A Theory of Social Interaction*; Stanford University Press: Stanford, CA, USA, 1988.
16. Burke, P.J. *Contemporary Social Psychological Theories*; Stanford University Press: Stanford, CA, USA, 2020.
17. Mikkelsen, K.; Stojanovska, L.; Polenakovic, M.; Bosevski, M.; Apostolopoulos, V. Exercise and mental health. *Maturitas* **2017**, *106*, 48–56. [CrossRef]
18. Campion, M.; Levita, L. Enhancing positive affect and divergent thinking abilities: Play some music and dance. *J. Posit. Psychol.* **2014**, *9*, 137–145. [CrossRef]
19. Koch, S.; Kunz, T.; Lykou, S.; Cruz, R. Effects of dance movement therapy and dance on health-related psychological outcomes: A meta-analysis. *Arts Psychother* **2014**, *41*, 46–64. [CrossRef]
20. Thompson, M. *Cultural Theory*; Routledge: New York, NY, USA, 2018.

21. Zhang, Z.; Pi, Z.; Liu, B. TROIKA: A general framework for heart rate monitoring using wrist-type photoplethysmographic signals during intensive physical exercise. *IEEE. Trans. Biomed.* **2015**, *62*, 522–531. [CrossRef]
22. Kim, J.; Lee, J.; Woo, J. Is heart rate measured by smartwatch during exercise reliable? Analysis of correlation and agreement between heart rates of Polar and smartwatch. *J. Korea Converg. Soc.* **2020**, *11*, 331–339.
23. Nieri, T.; Hughes, E. All about having fun: Women's experience of Zumba fitness. *Sociol. Sport J.* **2016**, *33*, 135–145. [CrossRef]
24. Luettgen, M.; Foster, C.; Doberstein, S.; Mikat, R.; Porcari, J. ZUMBA®: Is the "fitness-party" a good workout? *J. Sci. Med. Sport* **2012**, *11*, 357–358.
25. Riebe, D.; Ehrman, J.K.; Linguori, G.; Magal, M. (Eds.) *American College of Sports Medicine's Guidelines for Exercise Testing and Prescription*, 10th ed.; Kluwer: Philadelphia, PA, USA, 2017.
26. Donath, L.; Roth, R.; Hohn, Y.; Zahner, L.; Faude, O. The effects of Zumba training on cardiovascular and neuromuscular function in female college students. *Eur. J. Sport Sci.* **2014**, *14*, 569–577. [CrossRef]
27. Haghjoo, M.; Zar, A.; Hoseini, S.A. The Effect of 8 weeks Zumba Training on Women's Body Composition with Overweight. *Pars Jahrom Univ. Med Sci.* **2016**, *14*, 21–30. [CrossRef]
28. Lee, J.; Park, J.; Kim, Y.; Woo, M. Affective Change with Variations in Zumba Fitness Intensity as Measured by a Smartwatch. *Percept. Mot. Skills* **2021**, *128*, 2255–2278. [CrossRef]
29. Cugusi, L.; Wilson, B.; Serpe, R.; Medda, A.; Deidda, M.; Gabba, S.; Satta, G.; Chiappori, P.; Mercuro, G. Cardiovascular effects, body composition, quality of life and pain after a Zumba fitness program in Italian overweight women. *J. Sports Med. Phys. Fit.* **2016**, *56*, 328–335.
30. Norouzi, E.; Hosseini, F.; Vaezmosavi, M.; Gerber, M.; Puhse, U.; Brand, S. Zumba dancing and aerobic exercise can improve working memory, motor function, and depressive symptoms in female patients with Fibromyalgia. *Eur. J. Sport Sci.* **2020**, *20*, 981–991. [CrossRef]
31. Faul, F.; Erdfelder, E.; Buchner, A.; Lang, A.-G. Statistical power analyses using G*Power 3.1: Tests for correlation and regression analyses. *Behav. Res. Methods* **2009**, *41*, 1149–1160. [CrossRef]
32. Ministry of Culture, Sports and Tourism. *Development of Standards for National Fitness in Adulthood;* Ministry of Culture, Sports and Tourism: Sejong, Korea, 2010.
33. Ministry of Culture, Sports and Tourism. *Improvement of National Fitness 100 Evaluation Criteria;* Ministry of Culture, Sports and Tourism: Sejong, Korea, 2015.
34. Henriksen, A.; Haugen Mikalsen, M.; Woldaregay, A.Z.; Muzny, M.; Hartvigsen, G.; Hopstock, L.A.; Grimsgaard, S. Using Fitness Trackers and Smartwatches to Measure Physical Activity in Research: Analysis of Consumer Wrist-Worn Wearables. *J. Med. Internet Res.* **2018**, *20*, e110. [CrossRef] [PubMed]
35. Watson, D.; Clark, L.A. *The PANAS-X: Manual for the Positive and Negative Affect Schedule-Expanded Form;* University of Iowa: Iowa City, IA, USA, 1994.
36. Russell, J.A. A circumplex model of affect. *J. Pers. Soc. Psychol.* **1980**, *39*, 1161–1178. [CrossRef]
37. Russell, J.A. Core affect and the psychological construction of emotion. *Psychol. Rev.* **2003**, *110*, 145–172. [CrossRef] [PubMed]
38. Hardy, C.J.; Rejeski, W.J. Not what, but how one feels: The measurement of affect during exercise. *J. Psychol Sport Exerc.* **1989**, *11*, 304–317. [CrossRef]
39. Svebak, S.; Murgatroyd, S. Metamotivational dominance: A multimethod validation of reversal theory constructs. *J. Pers. Soc. Psychol.* **1985**, *48*, 107–116. [CrossRef]
40. Fox, S.M., III. Physical activity and the prevention of coronary heart disease. *Ann. Med. Res.* **1971**, *3*, 404–432. [CrossRef]
41. Garber, C.E.; Blissmer, B.; Deschenes, M.R.; Franklin, B.A.; Lamonte, M.J.; Lee, I.-M.; Nieman, D.C.; Swain, D.P. American College of Sports Medicine position stand. Quantity and quality of exercise for developing and maintaining cardiorespiratory, musculoskeletal, and neuromotor fitness in apparently healthy adults: Guidance for prescribing exercise. *Med. Sci. Sports Exerc.* **2011**, *43*, 1334–1359. [CrossRef] [PubMed]
42. Perez, B.; Greenwood-Robinson, M. *Zumba: Ditch the Workout, Join the Party! The Zumba Weight Loss Program;* Grand Central Life & Style: New York, NY, USA, 2014.
43. Yu, J.; Park, S. K-Pop Girl Group Dance Movement Classification Systems and Visualization Implementation. *Korean J. Danc.* **2019**, *19*, 25–36.
44. Ekkekakis, P.; Petruzzello, S.J. Acute aerobic exercise and affect. *Sports Med.* **1999**, *28*, 337–347. [CrossRef]
45. Busing, K.; West, C. Determining the relationship between physical fitness, gender, and life satisfaction. *SAGE Open.* **2016**, *6*, 1–5. [CrossRef]
46. Rezazadeh, A.; Talebi, N. Relationship Between Emotion Regulation and Health-Related of Physical Fitness in Tehran Firefighters. *Clin. Psychol. Personal.* **2021**. [CrossRef]
47. Lin, T.-W.; Kuo, Y.-M. Exercise Benefits Brain Function: The Monoamine Connection. *Brain Sci.* **2013**, *3*, 39–53. [CrossRef] [PubMed]
48. Melancon, M.; Lorrain, D.; Dionne, I. Exercise and sleep in aging: Emphasis on serotonin. *Pathol. Biol.* **2014**, *62*, 276–283. [CrossRef]
49. Klaperski, S.; von Dawans, B.; Heinrichs, M.; Fuchs, R. Effects of a 12-week endurance training program on the physiological response to psychosocial stress in men: A randomized controlled trial. *J. Behav. Med.* **2014**, *37*, 1118–1133. [CrossRef]

50. Childs, E.; de Wit, H. Regular exercise is associated with emotional resilience to acute stress in healthy adults. *Front. Physiol.* **2014**, *5*, 161. [CrossRef] [PubMed]
51. Strahler, J.; Fuchs, R.; Nater, U.M.; Klaperski, S. Impact of physical fitness on salivary stress markers in sedentary to low-active young to middle-aged men. *Psychoneuroendocrinology* **2016**, *68*, 14–19. [CrossRef]
52. Wood, C.J.; Clow, A.; Hucklebridge, F.; Law, R.; Smyth, N. Physical fitness and prior physical activity are both associated with less cortisol secretion during psychosocial stress. *Anxiety Stress Coping* **2018**, *31*, 135–145. [CrossRef] [PubMed]

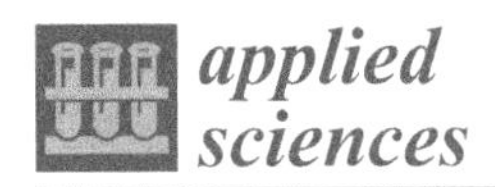

applied sciences

MDPI

Review

Bimanual Movements and Chronic Stroke Rehabilitation: Looking Back and Looking Forward

James H. Cauraugh [1,*] and Nyeonju Kang [2]

[1] Department of Applied Physiology and Kinesiology, University of Florida, Gainesville, FL 32611-8206, USA
[2] Division of Sport Science, Sport Science Institute, and Health Promotion Center, Incheon National University, Incheon 22012, Korea; nyunju@inu.ac.kr
* Correspondence: cauraugh@ufl.edu; Tel.: +1-352-294-1623

Abstract: Executing voluntary motor actions in the upper extremities after a stroke is frequently challenging and frustrating. Although spontaneous motor recovery can occur, reorganizing the activation of the primary motor cortex and supplementary motor area takes a considerable amount of time involving effective rehabilitation interventions. Based on motor control theory and experience-dependent neural plasticity, stroke protocols centered on bimanual movement coordination are generating considerable evidence in overcoming dysfunctional movements. Looking backward and forward in this comprehensive review, we discuss noteworthy upper extremity improvements reported in bimanual movement coordination studies including force generation. Importantly, the effectiveness of chronic stroke rehabilitation approaches that involve voluntary interlimb coordination principles look promising.

Keywords: chronic stroke; bimanual movement; bimanual force control; rehabilitation

Citation: Cauraugh, J.H.; Kang, N. Bimanual Movements and Chronic Stroke Rehabilitation: Looking Back and Looking Forward. *Appl. Sci.* **2021**, *11*, 10858. https://doi.org/10.3390/app112210858

Academic Editor: Redha Taiar

Received: 28 September 2021
Accepted: 16 November 2021
Published: 17 November 2021

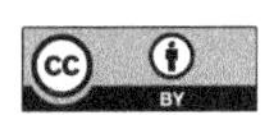

1. Introduction

Bimanual movement coordination has a long history and sound theoretical basis as an effective treatment to relearn dysfunctional motor actions caused by a stroke. Typical dysfunctional motor actions on the affected side of the body include weakness or partial paralysis. Planning and executing bimanual movements with an emphasis on simultaneously activating both limbs as a coordinative structure frequently facilitates progress toward motor recovery. Although the concept of bimanual movement coordination as a treatment for chronic stroke was first proposed over 60 years ago [1,2], the intervention has continued to develop, stimulating research and debate. This article will emphasize the rationale and evidence supporting bimanual movement coordination interventions as well as present persuasive arguments considering various rehabilitation treatment prescriptions.

When blood flow in the brain is disrupted by a focal neurological insult, mild to severe motor action dysfunctions become apparent on the contralateral side of the body. Granted, spontaneous motor action recovery can occur; however, a majority of the individuals (approximate 80–90%) who experienced a stroke must cope with hemiparesis [3]. Fortunately, dysfunctional motor actions are no longer viewed as permanent given the convincing neural plasticity evidence [4–8]. Even though Hebb postulated that synaptic plasticity was possible in 1949, the tendency of synapses and neuronal circuits to change because of activity took time to become accepted. Today, neural plasticity (i.e., brain changes that occur in response to experience-dependent challenges) and robust evidence supporting activity-based movements are primary components of multiple treatment protocols post-stroke [7–13]. Planning and executing simultaneous bimanual coordination actions are viable treatment protocols to minimize upper extremity motor dysfunctions post-stroke.

Recent studies on the contributions of the cerebral hemispheres involved in activity-based motor actions revealed focal areas active in excitation and inhibition [14]. Balancing activation of both hemispheres is still relevant to re-acquiring movements post-stroke.

Moreover, in a discussion of non-invasive brain stimulation protocols, Bestmann and colleagues [15,16] stated that the premotor cortex and supplementary motor cortex readily interact with targeted primary motor cortex areas generating motor action improvements. Supporting evidence favoring this argument was reported by Byblow and colleagues when they tested stroke individuals and found increased corticomotor excitability post bimanual symmetrical (mirror) movements [17]. Further, Liao and colleagues revealed post-stroke bimanual coordination benefits for severely impaired individuals when stimulating the contralesional dorsal premotor cortex, whereas facilitating the ipsilesional motor cortex improved coordination for individuals with mildly impaired upper extremities [18]. In summary, post-stroke bimanual movements are less dysfunctional after receiving brain activity modulation in the primary motor cortex as well as the premotor and supplementary cortex areas of both hemispheres [19–23]. This conclusion is consistent with Carson's comprehensive review article on neural control and bimanual arm interactions [24].

2. Chronic Stroke Rehabilitation

For chronic stroke rehabilitation, we are concerned with neural plasticity changes that occur during activity-based neural reorganization that occurs across time. The treatments are designed to re-acquire motor actions so that new and stable permanent memories for movements are created. Although there is consensus that intact brain areas may take over dysfunctional motor actions, specific details involving neural reorganization are still unclear. Granted, lesion location and extent contribute to reorganization, whereas rehabilitation frequency and intensity certainly facilitate the process. Rehabilitation specialists are experimenting with individually prescribed treatment protocols for focal neurological lesions of the motor system. An emerging theme is that neural networks closely aligned anatomically to the lesion site progressively adopt the functions of the damaged area over time and increased synaptic activity becomes apparent [7,8,10]. Indeed, Nudo [8] argued that recovering motor actions indicate waves of growth promotion and inhibition that modulate the adjacent intact tissue during the brain's self-repair processes.

2.1. Activity-Based Movements (Experience-Dependent Movements)

For maximum and lasting motor action benefits, stroke protocols should be founded on a sound theoretical framework based on motor learning and control principles [25,26]. Importantly, activity-based movements or experienced-dependent movements are sound stroke rehabilitation treatment protocols that have consistently expedited progress toward stroke recovery in the upper extremities [27–29]. Persuasive evidence comes from Sheahan, Franklin, and Wolpert [30] in a motor planning and execution experiment. Participants performed reaching movements through a force-field that perturbed movements. They found that motor planning and neural control enhanced movement learning by forming motor memories.

An implication for stroke interventions is that individuals should be actively involved in planning motor actions [31], and this includes both arms intentionally moving simultaneously. Combining motor planning and performing bimanual upper extremity movements highlights the basis for conducting activity-dependent movements to create new neural connections. Specifically, neural plasticity changes evolve from the Hebbian synapse rule that states that individual synaptic junctions respond to activity/use and inactivity/disuse [32–34]. Experience-dependent long-term modification of synaptic efficacy underlies motor memories in neural networks [30,35–37].

2.2. Bimanual Movement Interventions

Compelling evidence suggests that assimilation occurs between the left and right arms during neural control of symmetrical bimanual motor actions [24,38]. Promising findings on chronic stroke interventions have been identified when participants perform the same movement with both limbs. Further, producing the same forces on both arms with homologous muscles firing simultaneously post-stroke assists in making progress toward motor recovery. Early bimanual coordination or bimanual coordination studies consistently reported synchronization among effectors in concurrently performed movements [24,39–51]. Importantly, Bernstein's classic argument that both arms are centrally linked as a coordinative structure holds, and upper extremities function in a homologous coupling of muscle groups on both sides of the body [52].

A series of chronic stroke studies focused on bimanual movements executed concurrently and supplemented with neuromuscular-triggered electrical stimulation revealed consistent motor improvement findings. Manipulating treatment protocols centered on bimanual movements as well as EMG-triggered stimulation generates progress toward motor recovery in the upper extremities [21,38,53–58]. Positive experience-dependent and active stimulation findings include increased motor capabilities in short-term and longitudinal post-testing. Moreover, adding a proportional load to the non-paretic arm while requiring bimanual movements produced less dysfunctional motor actions in the impaired arm/hand. In a systematic review and meta-analysis on bimanual movement coordination (i.e., interlimb coordination) protocols post-stroke indicated that the chronic stroke groups improved performance while executing both synchronous and asynchronous bimanual movements [54]. Further, Whitall and colleagues found asynchronous support when they strapped the paretic and non-paretic arms to cars attached to a trackway and required participants to perform rhythmic alternating (asynchronous) bimanual movements [59].

3. Bimanual Kinematic and Kinetic Functions in Chronic Stroke

Motor impairments on one side of the upper body such as muscle weakness, spasticity, and loss of motor skills in the affected arm typically appear in patients with stroke [3]. Further, the increased asymmetrical motor functions between paretic and non-paretic arms interfere with bimanual movement control capabilities (e.g., bimanual performances and coordination) required for successful execution of activities of daily living [60,61]. For example, common post-stroke motor impairments include movement initiation and control on command as well as coordination problems during bimanual arm/hand reaching, moving objects, hand drawing, and finger tapping tasks [62–66]. According to motor control theory, movement kinetics are the primary components involved in activating motor actions [67–70]. As individuals post-stroke initiate or attempt to initiate arm movements, generating forces in the paretic arm are imperative. One way to facilitate this process or system is to require the non-paretic arm to initiate the same movement. Symmetrical motor performances are easier to execute than asymmetrical movements.

Kantak and colleagues suggested that estimating interlimb coordination is crucial for stroke motor rehabilitation because less cooperative upper limb movements post-stroke can increase motor reliance on the non-paretic arm compromising the efficiency of motor actions requiring both arms (e.g., opening the drawer with the non-paretic arm) [66]. Thus, investigating potential motor rehabilitation protocols for improving bimanual coordination functions is useful for facilitating progress toward motor recovery.

A recent meta-analysis study summarized specific patterns of bimanual movement and coordination deficits post-stroke [71]. Patients with stroke showed more interlimb kinematic and kinetic coordination impairments than age-matched healthy controls while executing asymmetrical movements with more difficult task goals such as asymmetric movement with independent goals and asymmetric parallel movements with a common goal for each hand [63,72]. These impairments were additionally observed in symmetric movement tasks when two hands targeted a common task goal. Bimanual movement tasks consisting of more challenging task constraints typically require more interactive behavioral communications between two arms with increased motor-related cortical activation across the primary motor area and supplementary motor areas [73,74]. Thus, unbalanced cortical activation and interhemispheric inhibition levels between hemispheres post-stroke may cause more impairments in bimanual movement and coordination with more difficult task goals [75]. Interestingly, meta-regression results indicated that deficits in bimanual coordination were significantly associated with increased time since stroke onset [71].

These findings indicate that despite relatively rapid recovery progress within six months post-stroke [76], bimanual movement control capabilities continue to be compromised in the chronic stage of motor recovery.

In addition to bimanual kinematic dysfunctions post-stroke, impairments in bimanual kinetic functions often appeared in patients with stroke. Kang and Cauraugh [77] conducted a comprehensive literature review that demonstrated potential deficits in bimanual force control capabilities in post-stroke individuals. While processing visual feedback displaying isometric forces produced by both hands and a targeted submaximal force level, stroke groups revealed less force accuracy (e.g., root mean squared error) and variability (e.g., coefficient of variation), indicating more erroneous and inconsistent force generation patterns during bimanual wrist extension and gripping force tasks [78–81]. Moreover, bimanual forces produced by participants post-stroke tended to be more regular (i.e., greater force regularity) as indicated by higher values of approximate entropy [79,82,83], and these patterns indicated decreased motor adaptability during force control tasks [84]. Asymmetrical muscular functions between the paretic and non-paretic hands as well as impaired sensorimotor processing may be responsible for lower submaximal bimanual force control performances from 5% to 50% of maximum voluntary contraction (MVC) [78,83].

Importantly, interlimb force coordination patterns were additionally impaired after stroke onset. Lodha and colleagues reported lower values of cross-correlation strength with increased time-lag as compared with age-matched controls during bimanual isometric wrist and fingers extension tasks [83]. These findings suggested that stroke may interfere with temporal coordination between paretic and non-paretic hands, and further non-paretic hands presumably modulated their forces to compensate for lacking forces generated by paretic hands during bimanual force control [81,85]. These deficits in interlimb coordination in individuals with stroke were additionally observed in dynamical force control tasks (e.g., force increment and decrement phases) [86]. Moreover, altered bimanual force coordination in patients with stroke were significantly associated with motor impairments as indicated by various clinical assessments (e.g., the Fugl–Meyer assessment and Pegboard assembly score) [81,82,86]. Proposed neurophysiological mechanisms underlying impairments abound for bimanual movements and bimanual coordination [39,40], including altered sensorimotor integration capabilities post-stroke such as online motor correction using simultaneous visual information [87]. Further, increased interhemispheric inhibition from the contralesional hemisphere typically suppresses cortical activation of the ipsilesional hemisphere, which may send biased efferent signals to the paretic and non-paretic arms, causing impaired interlimb coordination functions [73,88]. Indeed, changes in somatosensory feedback influenced by stroke appear to be a crucial reason in weakening interlimb coordination because prior studies showed more deficits in force coordination without a visual feedback condition for chronic stroke patients [79,89].

Beyond the altered bimanual motor control functions within a trial, recent studies explored changes in bimanual coordination strategies across multiple trials for post-stroke individuals. Sainburg and colleagues proposed the importance of bimanual motor synergies reflecting different cooperative behaviors between hands across multiple trials in stroke motor rehabilitation [43]. According to the uncontrolled manifold hypothesis [90–92], motor variability consists of two components: good and bad variability. During multiple trials of a bimanual force control task, the fundamental elements can include pairs of left and right mean forces within a trial. Good variability is the variance of fundamental elements projected on the uncontrolled manifold line that does not influence the stability of task performance (e.g., overall force accuracy across multiple trials). However, greater good variability indicates that the motor system produces more possible motor solutions (i.e., motor flexibility), whereas less good variability denotes that the motor system selects a more consistent motor solution (i.e., motor optimality). Bad variability is the variance of fundamental elements projected on the line orthogonal to the uncontrolled manifold line that does influence the stability of task performance. Increased bad variability impairs the stabilization of task performance across multiple trials. Taken together, given that the index of bimanual motor synergies is the proportion of good variability relative to bad variability, increased values of bimanual motor synergies across bimanual force control trials indicate better bimanual coordination strategies across trials contributing to overall task stabilization. In fact, Kang and Cauraugh [38] examined bimanual motor synergies in chronic stroke patients during bimanual force control tasks. The stroke group revealed less bimanual motor synergies than age-matched controls at 50% of MVC, and chronic stroke patients increased bad variability levels from 5% to 50% of MVC. These findings indicated that an impaired motor system post-stroke may compromise motor functions at the execution level (i.e., within a trial) as well as planning level (i.e., between trials). Thus, future stroke motor interventions should examine the effects of interactive motor actions between the paretic and non-paretic arms.

4. Looking Forward

What is on the horizon for bimanual movement interventions and chronic stroke rehabilitation? Rehabilitation interventions should aim for maximum recovery of function through motor learning improvements on the hemiplegic side [22]. Applying non-invasive brain stimulation (NIBS) in addition to motor training may be an attractive treatment protocol for improving bimanual coordination function post-stroke. Pixa and Pollak [93] suggested potential effects of transcranial direct current stimulation (tDCS), one of the NIBS protocols, on bimanual motor skills in heathy individuals. Two tDCS stimulations consist of anodal tDCS that may potentially increase cortical excitability and cathodal tDCS that may potentially suppress cortical excitability. Specific tDCS protocols for facilitating bimanual motor function improvements involved (a) anodal tDCS on the primary motor cortex (M1) of the ipsilesional hemisphere and cathodal tDCS on M1 of the contralesional hemisphere and (b) anodal tDCS on M1 of bimanual hemispheres [94–96]. Theoretically, these tDCS protocols are expected to be effective for re-balancing brain activations between affected and unaffected hemispheres, contributing to functional improvements in bimanual actions (e.g., bimanual typing performance and Perdue pegboard test). In testing chronic stroke patients, many prior studies reported transient and sustained treatment effects of tDCS protocols on unilateral paretic arm functions [22,97,98], whereas potential tDCS effects on bimanual motor functions are still insufficient. A limited number of studies revealed that bihemispheric tDCS in addition to conventional physical therapy improved interlimb coordinative skills in patients with stroke [99,100].

Beyond the interhemispheric competition model emphasizing the balanced excitatory and inhibitory activations between hemispheres post-stroke via tDCS [20,101], a recent approach proposed the bimodal balance-recovery model integrating both vicariation and interhemispheric competition approaches [75]. Intriguingly, this model posited that the vicariation model, assuming the important role of the unaffected hemisphere for functional recovery of the paretic limbs, may be beneficial for stroke patients with lower structure reserve (e.g., more severe and wide ranges of brain lesion), whereas the interhemispheric competition model may be effective for stroke patients with higher structure reserve (e.g., more recovered brain regions). Based on this model, applying cathodal tDCS suppressing the contralesional hemisphere may decrease treatment effects on motor recovery of patients with severe brain damages and less recovered brain functions (e.g., acute and subacute phases). In fact, several meta-analytic findings evidenced that tDCS protocols including cathodal tDCS on the contralesional hemisphere revealed overall significant positive effects on motor recovery, whereas this protocol failed to show functional improvements in the paretic arms of the acute and subacute patients with stroke [102,103]. These findings support a proposition that bihemispheric tDCS protocols should be individualized based on either the severity or the recovery state of affected brain regions. For example, applying anodal tDCS on the primary motor cortex of bimanual hemispheres may be more effective for improving bimanual motor functions in patients with acute and subacute patients [104].

One caveat about tDCS protocols concerns the general brain assumptions necessary to ensure individual treatment benefits. That is, tDCS stimulation effects that are dose-controlled according to electrode size, location placement, and stimulus intensity will minimize the trial-and-error effect frequently seen with so many stroke-rehabilitation protocols [105]. Establishing accepted procedures in administering tDCS should lead to individualized dose-controlled treatments [98]. Further, standardizing tDCS protocols for chronic stroke intervention must include when and duration of the anodal and cathodal stimulation combinations [106]. Questions on the optimal stimulation time are still being debated. Should chronic stroke individuals receive 20–30 min of tDCS before performing bimanual movement training or should 20–30 min of stimulation occur simultaneously with bimanual movements?

Moreover, developing isometric rehabilitation programs may be a viable option for facilitating functional recovery of the paretic arm. Given that isometric contraction requires no dynamic movements, patients with stroke can safely participate in the isometric training regardless of their muscle weakness and spasticity in the paretic arms as prior findings suggested [107–109]. Moreover, Kang and colleagues raised a possibility that bimanual actions transiently increased motor functions in the paretic arms by demonstrating greater maximal and submaximal mean forces and less force variability and regularity produced by the paretic arm during bimanual force control tasks than those during unimanual force control tasks [110,111]. These findings indicated that applying bimanual isometric training protocols can be an additional effective approach to improvements in acquiring coordinative motor skills post-stroke.

To facilitate motor recovery progress post-stroke, pharmacological therapies can be viable alternatives [13,112]. For example, a meta-analysis study reported that the serotonin reuptake inhibitor (SSRI) fluoxetine improved motor recovery in acute and subacute patients (less than 3 months since stroke) [113]. Potentially, the SSRI fluoxetine may be beneficial for motor improvements via the facilitation of neurogenesis and anti-inflammatory neuroprotection and enhancing cerebral blood flow according to the findings from animal models [114]. Importantly, the appropriate timing of these pharmacological treatments would be within first three months since the stroke because this period presumably increases a possibility of interactive effects between pharmacological treatments and spontaneous recovery maximizing motor rehabilitation. Despite controversial treatment effects on stroke patients with increased time since the stroke (e.g., >6 months), pharmacological interventions would be an additional option for improving bimanual motor functions in chronic patients.

5. Summary

The current evidence on experience-dependent neural changes is becoming integrated in rehabilitation protocols focused on individuals in the chronic stroke stage of recovery (Figure 1). Indeed, accumulated findings on bimanual movements training indicate an effective and efficient intervention to address post-stroke motor dysfunctions. Practicing bimanual coordination movements improves the motor capabilities on the impaired side of the upper extremity. Specifically, four sets of evidence form a converging operations conclusion that bimanual coordination movement training treatments are positive: (a) a primer for a typical treatment protocol, which includes activating the muscles involved in the treatment before beginning the stroke protocol; (b) in conjunction with neuromuscular-triggered electrical stimulation; (c) while executing rhythmic alternating movements; and (d) robotic guided rehabilitation [20,53,115–117].

Concerning the neural networks and brain areas involved in changing the severity of motor dysfunctions, science has made important advances in understanding the interactions among brain areas [118–121]. However, exact details on the distributed neural networks connecting the cortical and subcortical brain areas active during voluntary motor actions are still being explored. Consistent with Baddeley's elegant discussion of the concept of working memory evolving with the addition of new empirical findings, neural plasticity and distributed networks interacting with various brain mechanisms are still evolving [122,123].

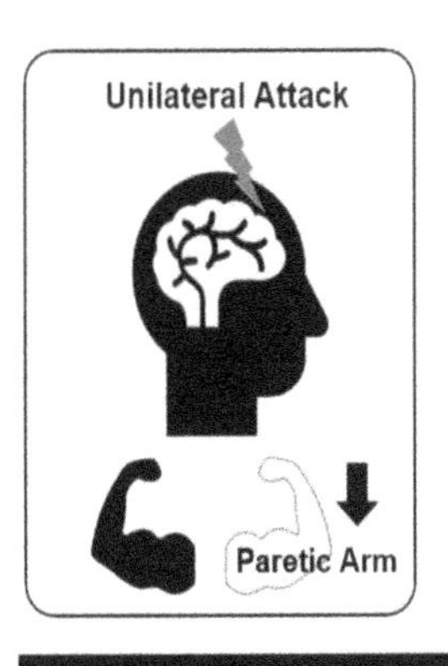
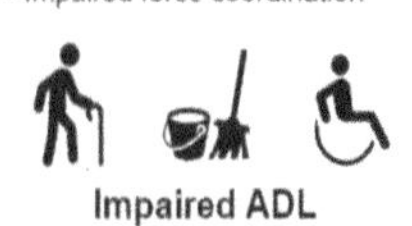
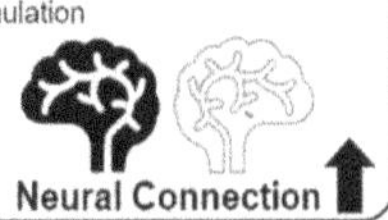

Figure 1. Progress toward stroke motor recovery using bimanual motor training.

Together, the current empirical bimanual movement training findings present a persuasive alternative to unilateral rehabilitation post-stroke. The time has come to select bimanual coordination as a sound theoretical basis for making progress toward motor recovery post-stroke and abandon one arm protocols. Logical and convincing arguments on motor actions involved in planning and executing challenging bimanual movements, perhaps with an assistive device (e.g., neuromuscular electrical stimulation or robotic manipulandum) included in the intervention, will advance our understanding of effective and efficient interventions. Based on the accumulated evidence [54,77,86,124,125], chronic post-stroke individuals who are prescribed experience-dependent treatments that include bimanual coordinated movements will display fewer impaired motor actions.

Granted, comprehensive post-stroke rehabilitation protocols with the explicit intention of making progress toward motor recovery should closely follow the guidelines recommended by the American Heart Association [32] as well as England's Queen Square Upper Limb Neurorehabilitation Program [126]. As Cauraugh and Summers stated in 2005, the efficacy and effectiveness of post-stroke bimanual movement interventions will advance rapidly when groups of individuals are matched according to lesion location, lesion size, and impairment severity [50]. Individualized post-stroke rehabilitation prescriptions are steps in the right direction.

Author Contributions: Conceptualization, J.H.C. and N.K.; methodology, J.H.C. and N.K.; data curation, J.H.C. and N.K.; writing—original draft preparation, J.H.C. and N.K.; writing—review and editing, J.H.C. and N.K.; All authors have read and agreed to the published version of the manuscript.

Funding: This research received no external funding.

Institutional Review Board Statement: Not applicable.

Informed Consent Statement: Not applicable.

Data Availability Statement: Not applicable.

Conflicts of Interest: The authors declare no conflict of interest.

References

1. Rose, D.K.; Winstein, C.J. Bimanual training after stroke: Are two hands better than one? *Top. Stroke Rehabil.* **2004**, *11*, 20–30. [CrossRef] [PubMed]
2. Rose, D.K.; Winstein, C.J. The co-ordination of bimanual rapid aiming movements following stroke. *Clin. Rehabil.* **2005**, *19*, 452–462. [CrossRef]

3. Virani, S.S.; Alonso, A.; Aparicio, H.J.; Benjamin, E.J.; Bittencourt, M.S.; Callaway, C.W.; Carson, A.P.; Chamberlain, A.M.; Cheng, S.; Delling, F.N.; et al. Heart disease and stroke statistics-2021 update: A report from the american heart association. *Circulation* **2021**, *143*, e254–e743. [CrossRef]
4. Hallett, M.; Di Iorio, R.; Rossini, P.M.; Park, J.E.; Chen, R.; Celnik, P.; Strafella, A.P.; Matsumoto, H.; Ugawa, Y. Contribution of transcranial magnetic stimulation to assessment of brain connectivity and networks. *Clin. Neurophysiol.* **2017**, *128*, 2125–2139. [CrossRef] [PubMed]
5. Buch, E.R.; Santarnecchi, E.; Antal, A.; Born, J.; Celnik, P.A.; Classen, J.; Gerloff, C.; Hallett, M.; Hummel, F.C.; Nitsche, M.A.; et al. Effects of tDCS on motor learning and memory formation: A consensus and critical position paper. *Clin. Neurophysiol.* **2017**, *128*, 589–603. [CrossRef] [PubMed]
6. Buch, E.R.; Liew, S.L.; Cohen, L.G. Plasticity of sensorimotor networks: Multiple overlapping mechanisms. *Neuroscientist* **2017**, *23*, 185–196. [CrossRef]
7. Nudo, R.J. Mechanisms for recovery of motor function following cortical damage. *Curr. Opin. Neurobiol.* **2006**, *16*, 638–644. [CrossRef]
8. Nudo, R.J. Plasticity. *NeuroRx* **2006**, *3*, 420–427. [CrossRef]
9. Nishibe, M.; Urban, E.T., 3rd; Barbay, S.; Nudo, R.J. Rehabilitative training promotes rapid motor recovery but delayed motor map reorganization in a rat cortical ischemic infarct model. *Neurorehabil. Neural Repair* **2015**, *29*, 472–482. [CrossRef]
10. Nudo, R.J. Rehabilitation: Boost for movement. *Nature* **2015**, *527*, 314–315. [CrossRef] [PubMed]
11. Barbay, S.; Guggenmos, D.J.; Nishibe, M.; Nudo, R.J. Motor representations in the intact hemisphere of the rat are reduced after repetitive training of the impaired forelimb. *Neurorehabil. Neural Repair* **2013**, *27*, 381–384. [CrossRef] [PubMed]
12. Cramer, S.C. Stroke recovery: How the computer reprograms itself. Neuronal plasticity: The key to stroke recovery. Kananskis, alberta, canada, 19–22 march 2000. *Mol. Med. Today* **2000**, *6*, 301–303. [CrossRef]
13. Cramer, S.C.; Sur, M.; Dobkin, B.H.; O'Brien, C.; Sanger, T.D.; Trojanowski, J.Q.; Rumsey, J.M.; Hicks, R.; Cameron, J.; Chen, D.; et al. Harnessing neuroplasticity for clinical applications. *Brain* **2011**, *134*, 1591–1609. [CrossRef] [PubMed]
14. Cohen, L.G.; Hallett, M. Neural plasticity and recover of function. In *Handbook of Neurological Rehabilitation Greenwood, R.J., Barnes, M.P., McMillan, T.M., Ward, C.D., Eds.*; Psychology Press: Hove, UK, 2003; pp. 99–111.
15. Bestmann, S.; Duque, J. Transcranial magnetic stimulation: Decomposing the processes underlying action preparation. *Neuroscientist* **2016**, *22*, 392–405. [CrossRef]
16. Bestmann, S.; de Berker, A.O.; Bonaiuto, J. Understanding the behavioural consequences of noninvasive brain stimulation. *Trends Cogn. Sci.* **2015**, *19*, 13–20. [CrossRef]
17. Byblow, W.D.; Stinear, C.M.; Smith, M.C.; Bjerre, L.; Flaskager, B.K.; McCambridge, A.B. Mirror symmetric bimanual movement priming can increase corticomotor excitability and enhance motor learning. *PLoS ONE* **2012**, *7*, e33882.
18. Liao, W.W.; Whitall, J.; Wittenberg, G.F.; Barton, J.E.; Waller, S.M. Not all brain regions are created equal for improving bimanual coordination in individuals with chronic stroke. *Clin. Neurophysiol.* **2019**, *130*, 1218–1230. [CrossRef] [PubMed]
19. Butefisch, C.M.; Wessling, M.; Netz, J.; Seitz, R.J.; Homberg, V. Relationship between interhemispheric inhibition and motor cortex excitability in subacute stroke patients. *Neurorehabil. Neural Repair* **2008**, *22*, 4–21. [CrossRef]
20. Bao, S.C.; Khan, A.; Song, R.; Kai-Yu Tong, R. Rewiring the lesioned brain: Electrical stimulation for post-stroke motor restoration. *J. Stroke* **2020**, *22*, 47–63. [CrossRef]
21. Cauraugh, J.H.; Kim, S.B.; Duley, A. Coupled bilateral movements and active neuromuscular stimulation: Intralimb transfer evidence during bimanual aiming. *Neurosci. Lett.* **2005**, *382*, 39–44. [CrossRef]
22. Kang, N.; Summers, J.J.; Cauraugh, J.H. Transcranial direct current stimulation facilitates motor learning post-stroke: A systematic review and meta-analysis. *J. Neurol. Neurosurg. Psychiatry* **2016**, *87*, 345–355. [CrossRef]
23. Bradnam, L.V.; Stinear, C.M.; Barber, P.A.; Byblow, W.D. Contralesional hemisphere control of the proximal paretic upper limb following stroke. *Cereb. Cortex* **2012**, *22*, 2662–2671. [CrossRef] [PubMed]
24. Carson, R.G. Neural pathways mediating bilateral interactions between the upper limbs. *Brain Res. Rev.* **2005**, *49*, 641–662. [CrossRef]
25. Hidaka, Y.; Han, C.E.; Wolf, S.L.; Winstein, C.J.; Schweighofer, N. Use it and improve it or lose it: Interactions between arm function and use in humans post-stroke. *PLoS Comput. Biol.* **2012**, *8*, e1002343. [CrossRef] [PubMed]
26. Winstein, C.J.; Requejo, P.S.; Zelinski, E.M.; Mulroy, S.J.; Crimmins, E.M. A transformative subfield in rehabilitation science at the nexus of new technologies, aging, and disability. *Front. Psychol.* **2012**, *3*, 340. [CrossRef]
27. Hallett, M. Functional reorganization after lesions of the human brain: Studies with transcranial magnetic stimulation. *Rev. Neurol.* **2001**, *157*, 822–826. [PubMed]
28. Ziemann, U.; Muellbacher, W.; Hallett, M.; Cohen, L.G. Modulation of practice-dependent plasticity in human motor cortex. *Brain* **2001**, *124*, 1171–1181. [CrossRef]
29. Hallett, M. Plasticity of the human motor cortex and recovery from stroke. *Brain Res. Rev.* **2001**, *36*, 169–174. [CrossRef]
30. Sheahan, H.R.; Franklin, D.W.; Wolpert, D.M. Motor planning, not execution, separates motor memories. *Neuron* **2016**, *92*, 773–779. [CrossRef]
31. Dean, P.J.; Seiss, E.; Sterr, A. Motor planning in chronic upper-limb hemiparesis: Evidence from movement-related potentials. *PLoS ONE* **2012**, *7*, e44558.

32. Winstein, C.J.; Stein, J.; Arena, R.; Bates, B.; Cherney, L.R.; Cramer, S.C.; Deruyter, F.; Eng, J.J.; Fisher, B.; Harvey, R.L.; et al. Guidelines for adult stroke rehabilitation and recovery: A guideline for healthcare professionals from the american heart association/american stroke association. *Stroke* **2016**, *47*, e98–e169. [CrossRef] [PubMed]
33. Coupar, F.; Van Wijck, F.; Morris, J.; Pollock, A.; Langhorne, P. Simultaneous bilateral training for improving arm function after stroke. *Cochrane Database Syst. Rev.* **2007**, *14*, CD006432.
34. Cramer, S.C. Repairing the human brain after stroke. II. Restorative therapies. *Ann. Neurol.* **2008**, *63*, 549–560. [CrossRef]
35. Bear, M.F.; Connors, B.W.; Paradiso, M.A. *Neuroscience: Exploring the Brain*, 2nd ed.; Lippincott Williams & Wilkins: Baltimore, MD, USA, 2001.
36. Celnik, P.A.; Cohen, L.G. Modulation of motor function and cortical plasticity in health and disease. *Restor. Neurol. Neurosci.* **2004**, *22*, 261–268.
37. Wolters, A.; Sandbrink, F.; Schlottmann, A.; Kunesch, E.; Stefan, K.; Cohen, L.G.; Benecke, R.; Classen, J. A temporally asymmetric hebbian rule governing plasticity in the human motor cortex. *J. Neurophysiol.* **2003**, *89*, 2339–2345. [CrossRef]
38. Kang, N.; Cauraugh, J.H. Bilateral synergy as an index of force coordination in chronic stroke. *Exp. Brain Res.* **2017**, *235*, 1501–1509. [CrossRef]
39. Swinnen, S.P. Intermanual coordination: From behavioural principles to neural-network interactions. *Nat. Rev. Neurosci.* **2002**, *3*, 348–359. [CrossRef] [PubMed]
40. Swinnen, S.P.; Wenderoth, N. Two hands, one brain: Cognitive neuroscience of bimanual skill. *Trends Cogn. Sci.* **2004**, *8*, 18–25. [CrossRef]
41. Summers, J.J.; Kagerer, F.A.; Garry, M.I.; Hiraga, C.Y.; Loftus, A.; Cauraugh, J.H. Bilateral and unilateral movement training on upper limb function in chronic stroke patients: A TMS study. *J. Neurol. Sci.* **2007**, *252*, 76–82. [CrossRef]
42. Summers, J.J.; Byblow, W.D.; Bysouth-Young, D.F.; Semjen, A. Bimanual circle drawing during secondary task loading. *Mot. Control* **1998**, *2*, 106–113. [CrossRef] [PubMed]
43. Sainburg, R.; Good, D.; Przybyla, A. Bilateral synergy: A framework for post-stroke rehabilitation. *J. Neurol. Transl. Neurosci.* **2013**, *1*, 1–14.
44. Mani, S.; Mutha, P.K.; Przybyla, A.; Haaland, K.Y.; Good, D.C.; Sainburg, R.L. Contralesional motor deficits after unilateral stroke reflect hemisphere-specific control mechanisms. *Brain* **2013**, *136*, 1288–1303. [CrossRef]
45. Mutha, P.K.; Haaland, K.Y.; Sainburg, R.L. Rethinking motor lateralization: Specialized but complementary mechanisms for motor control of each arm. *PLoS ONE* **2013**, *8*, e58582.
46. Maenza, C.; Good, D.C.; Winstein, C.J.; Wagstaff, D.A.; Sainburg, R.L. Functional deficits in the less-impaired arm of stroke survivors depend on hemisphere of damage and extent of paretic arm impairment. *Neurorehabilit. Neural Repair* **2020**, *34*, 39–50. [CrossRef]
47. Stinear, J.W.; Byblow, W.D. Rhythmic bilateral movement training modulates corticomotor excitability and enhances upper limb motricity poststroke: A pilot study. *J. Clin. Neurophysiol.* **2004**, *21*, 124–131. [CrossRef]
48. Stinear, C.M.; Fleming, M.K.; Barber, P.A.; Byblow, W.D. Lateralization of motor imagery following stroke. *Clin. Neurophysiol.* **2007**, *118*, 1794–1801. [CrossRef]
49. Swinnen, S.P.; Duysens, J. (Eds.) *Neuro-Behavioral Deterrminants of Interlimb Coordination: A Multidisciplinary Approach*; Kluwer Academic Publishers: Norwell, MA, USA, 2004.
50. Cauraugh, J.H.; Summers, J.J. Neural plasticity and bilateral movements: A rehabilitation approach for chronic stroke. *Prog. Neurobiol.* **2005**, *75*, 309–320. [CrossRef]
51. Latash, M.L. *Synergy*; Oxford University Press: New York, NY, USA, 2008.
52. Bernstein, N. *The Co-Ordination and Regulation of Movements*; Pergamon Press: Oxford, UK, 1967.
53. Cauraugh, J.H.; Kim, S.B.; Summers, J.J. Chronic stroke longitudinal motor improvements: Cumulative learning evidence found in the upper extremity. *Cerebrovasc. Dis.* **2008**, *25*, 115–121. [CrossRef] [PubMed]
54. Cauraugh, J.H.; Lodha, N.; Naik, S.K.; Summers, J.J. Bilateral movement training and stroke motor recovery progress: A structured review and meta-analysis. *Hum. Mov. Sci.* **2010**, *29*, 853–870. [CrossRef] [PubMed]
55. Kang, N.; Roberts, L.M.; Aziz, C.; Cauraugh, J.H. Age-related deficits in bilateral motor synergies and force coordination. *BMC Geriatr.* **2019**, *19*, 287. [CrossRef] [PubMed]
56. Chen, R.; Cohen, L.G.; Hallett, M. Nervous system reorganization following injury. *Neuroscience* **2002**, *111*, 761–773. [CrossRef]
57. Cauraugh, J.H.; Coombes, S.A.; Lodha, N.; Naik, S.K.; Summers, J.J. Upper extremity improvements in chronic stroke: Coupled bilateral load training. *Restor. Neurol. Neurosci.* **2009**, *27*, 17–25. [CrossRef]
58. Cauraugh, J.H.; Naik, S.K.; Lodha, N.; Coombes, S.A.; Summers, J.J. Long-term rehabilitation for chronic stroke arm movements: A randomized controlled trial. *Clin. Rehabil.* **2011**, *25*, 1086–1096. [CrossRef]
59. Whitall, J.; McCombe Waller, S.; Silver, K.H.; Macko, R.F. Repetitive bilateral arm training with rhythmic auditory cueing improves motor function in chronic hemiparetic stroke. *Stroke* **2000**, *31*, 2390–2395. [CrossRef]
60. Sleimen-Malkoun, R.; Temprado, J.J.; Thefenne, L.; Berton, E. Bimanual training in stroke: How do coupling and symmetry-breaking matter? *BMC Neurol.* **2011**, *25*, 11. [CrossRef]
61. Ranganathan, R.; Gebara, R.; Andary, M.; Sylvain, J. Chronic stroke survivors show task-dependent modulation of motor variability during bimanual coordination. *J. Neurophysiol.* **2019**, *121*, 756–763. [CrossRef]

62. Kilbreath, S.L.; Crosbie, J.; Canning, C.G.; Lee, M.J. Inter-limb coordination in bimanual reach-to-grasp following stroke. *Disabil. Rehabil.* **2006**, *28*, 1435–1443. [CrossRef] [PubMed]
63. Kantak, S.; McGrath, R.; Zahedi, N. Goal conceptualization and symmetry of arm movements affect bimanual coordination in individuals after stroke. *Neurosci. Lett.* **2016**, *626*, 86–93. [CrossRef] [PubMed]
64. Lewis, G.N.; Byblow, W.D. Bimanual coordination dynamics in poststroke hemiparetics. *J. Mot. Behav.* **2004**, *36*, 174–188. [CrossRef] [PubMed]
65. Wu, C.Y.; Chou, S.H.; Kuo, M.Y.; Chen, C.L.; Lu, T.W.; Fu, Y.C. Effects of object size on intralimb and interlimb coordination during a bimanual prehension task in patients with left cerebral vascular accidents. *Mot. Control* **2008**, *12*, 296–310. [CrossRef]
66. Kantak, S.; Jax, S.; Wittenberg, G. Bimanual coordination: A missing piece of arm rehabilitation after stroke. *Restor. Neurol. Neurosci.* **2017**, *35*, 347–364. [CrossRef]
67. Kelso, J.A.S.; Stelmach, G.E. Central and peripheral mechanisms in motor control. In *Motor Control: Issues and Trends*; Academic Press: New York, NY, USA, 1976; pp. 1–40.
68. Georgopoulos, A.P. Behavioral and neural aspects of motor topology: Following bernstein's thread. In *Progress in Motor Control: Structure-Function Relations in Voluntary Movements*; Human Kinetics: Champaign, IL, USA, 2002.
69. Enoka, R.M. *Neuromechanics of Human Movement*, 4th ed.; Human Kinetics: Champaign, IL, USA, 2008.
70. Krakauer, J.W.; Ghez, C. Voluntary movement. In *Principles of Neural Science*, 4th ed.; McGraw Hill: New York, NY, USA, 2006.
71. Kim, R.K.; Kang, N. Bimanual coordination functions between paretic and nonparetic arms: A systematic review and meta-analysis. *J. Stroke Cerebrovasc. Dis.* **2020**, *29*, 104544. [CrossRef]
72. Rose, D.K.; Winstein, C.J. Temporal coupling is more robust than spatial coupling: An investigation of interlimb coordination after stroke. *J. Mot. Behav.* **2013**, *45*, 313–324. [CrossRef]
73. Tazoe, T.; Sasada, S.; Sakamoto, M.; Komiyama, T. Modulation of interhemispheric interactions across symmetric and asymmetric bimanual force regulations. *Eur. J. Neurosci.* **2013**, *37*, 96–104. [CrossRef]
74. Sadato, N.; Yonekura, Y.; Waki, A.; Yamada, H.; Ishii, Y. Role of the supplementary motor area and the right premotor cortex in the coordination of bimanual finger movements. *J. Neurosci.* **1997**, *17*, 9667–9674. [CrossRef] [PubMed]
75. Di Pino, G.; Pellegrino, G.; Assenza, G.; Capone, F.; Ferreri, F.; Formica, D.; Ranieri, F.; Tombini, M.; Ziemann, U.; Rothwell, J.C.; et al. Modulation of brain plasticity in stroke: A novel model for neurorehabilitation. *Nat. Rev. Neurol.* **2014**, *10*, 597–608. [CrossRef] [PubMed]
76. Meyer, S.; Verheyden, G.; Brinkmann, N.; Dejaeger, E.; De Weerdt, W.; Feys, H.; Gantenbein, A.R.; Jenni, W.; Laenen, A.; Lincoln, N.; et al. Functional and motor outcome 5 years after stroke is equivalent to outcome at 2 months: Follow-up of the collaborative evaluation of rehabilitation in stroke across europe. *Stroke* **2015**, *46*, 1613–1619. [CrossRef]
77. Kang, N.; Cauraugh, J.H. Force control in chronic stroke. *Neurosci. Biobehav. Rev.* **2015**, *52*, 38–48. [CrossRef] [PubMed]
78. Kang, N.; Cauraugh, J.H. Bimanual force variability and chronic stroke: Asymmetrical hand control. *PLoS ONE* **2014**, *9*, e101817. [CrossRef]
79. Kang, N.; Cauraugh, J.H. Bimanual force variability in chronic stroke: With and without visual information. *Neurosci. Lett.* **2015**, *587*, 41–45. [CrossRef] [PubMed]
80. Patel, P.; Lodha, N. Dynamic bimanual force control in chronic stroke: Contribution of non-paretic and paretic hands. *Exp. Brain Res.* **2019**, *237*, 2123–2133. [CrossRef]
81. Lai, C.H.; Sung, W.H.; Chiang, S.L.; Lu, L.H.; Lin, C.H.; Tung, Y.C.; Lin, C.H. Bimanual coordination deficits in hands following stroke and their relationship with motor and functional performance. *J. Neuroeng. Rehabil.* **2019**, *16*, 101. [CrossRef] [PubMed]
82. Lodha, N.; Patten, C.; Coombes, S.A.; Cauraugh, J.H. Bimanual force control strategies in chronic stroke: Finger extension versus power grip. *Neuropsychologia* **2012**, *50*, 2536–2545. [CrossRef] [PubMed]
83. Lodha, N.; Coombes, S.A.; Cauraugh, J.H. Bimanual isometric force control: Asymmetry and coordination evidence post stroke. *Clin. Neurophysiol.* **2012**, *123*, 787–795. [CrossRef] [PubMed]
84. Hu, X.; Newell, K.M. Aging, visual information, and adaptation to task asymmetry in bimanual force coordination. *J. Appl. Physiol. (1985)* **2011**, *111*, 1671–1680. [CrossRef]
85. Alberts, J.L.; Wolf, S.L. The use of kinetics as a marker for manual dexterity after stroke and stroke recovery. *Top. Stroke Rehabil.* **2009**, *16*, 223–236. [CrossRef]
86. Patel, P.; Lodha, N. Functional implications of impaired bimanual force coordination in chronic stroke. *Neurosci. Lett.* **2020**, *738*, 135387. [CrossRef]
87. Ridderikhoff, A.; Peper, C.L.; Beek, P.J. Unraveling interlimb interactions underlying bimanual coordination. *J. Neurophysiol.* **2005**, *94*, 3112–3125. [CrossRef]
88. Liuzzi, G.; Horniss, V.; Zimerman, M.; Gerloff, C.; Hummel, F.C. Coordination of uncoupled bimanual movements by strictly timed interhemispheric connectivity. *J. Neurosci.* **2011**, *31*, 9111–9117. [CrossRef]
89. Torre, K.; Hammami, N.; Metrot, J.; van Dokkum, L.; Coroian, F.; Mottet, D.; Amri, M.; Laffont, I. Somatosensory-related limitations for bimanual coordination after stroke. *Neurorehabil. Neural Repair* **2013**, *27*, 507–515. [CrossRef]
90. Latash, M.L.; Scholz, J.P.; Schoner, G. Motor control strategies revealed in the structure of motor variability. *Exerc. Sport Sci. Rev.* **2002**, *30*, 26–31. [CrossRef]
91. Latash, M.L.; Scholz, J.F.; Danion, F.; Schoner, G. Structure of motor variability in marginally redundant multifinger force production tasks. *Exp. Brain Res.* **2001**, *141*, 153–165. [CrossRef]

92. Scholz, J.P.; Schoner, G. The uncontrolled manifold concept: Identifying control variables for a functional task. *Exp. Brain Res.* **1999**, *126*, 289–306. [CrossRef] [PubMed]
93. Pixa, N.H.; Pollok, B. Effects of tDCS on bimanual motor skills: A brief review. *Front. Behav. Neurosci.* **2018**, *12*, 63. [CrossRef] [PubMed]
94. Gomes-Osman, J.; Field-Fote, E.C. Bihemispheric anodal corticomotor stimulation using transcranial direct current stimulation improves bimanual typing task performance. *J. Mot. Behav.* **2013**, *45*, 361–367. [CrossRef] [PubMed]
95. Pixa, N.H.; Steinberg, F.; Doppelmayr, M. Effects of high-definition anodal transcranial direct current stimulation applied simultaneously to both primary motor cortices on bimanual sensorimotor performance. *Front. Behav. Neurosci.* **2017**, *11*, 130. [CrossRef]
96. Furuya, S.; Klaus, M.; Nitsche, M.A.; Paulus, W.; Altenmuller, E. Ceiling effects prevent further improvement of transcranial stimulation in skilled musicians. *J. Neurosci.* **2014**, *34*, 13834–13839. [CrossRef]
97. Tedesco Triccas, L.; Burridge, J.H.; Hughes, A.M.; Pickering, R.M.; Desikan, M.; Rothwell, J.C.; Verheyden, G. Multiple sessions of transcranial direct current stimulation and upper extremity rehabilitation in stroke: A review and meta-analysis. *Clin. Neurophysiol.* **2016**, *127*, 946–955. [CrossRef]
98. Van Hoornweder, S.; Vanderzande, L.; Bloemers, E.; Verstraelen, S.; Depestele, S.; Cuypers, K.; Dun, K.V.; Strouwen, C.; Meesen, R. The effects of transcranial direct current stimulation on upper-limb function post-stroke: A meta-analysis of multiple-session studies. *Clin. Neurophysiol.* **2021**, *132*, 1897–1918. [CrossRef]
99. Doost, M.Y.; Orban de Xivry, J.J.; Herman, B.; Vanthournhout, L.; Riga, A.; Bihin, B.; Jamart, J.; Laloux, P.; Raymackers, J.M.; Vandermeeren, Y. Learning a bimanual cooperative skill in chronic stroke under noninvasive brain stimulation: A randomized controlled trial. *Neurorehabil. Neural Repair* **2019**, *33*, 486–498. [CrossRef]
100. Middleton, A.; Fritz, S.L.; Liuzzo, D.M.; Newman-Norlund, R.; Herter, T.M. Using clinical and robotic assessment tools to examine the feasibility of pairing tDCS with upper extremity physical therapy in patients with stroke and TBI: A consideration-of-concept pilot study. *NeuroRehabilitation* **2014**, *35*, 741–754. [CrossRef] [PubMed]
101. Nowak, D.A.; Grefkes, C.; Ameli, M.; Fink, G.R. Interhemispheric competition after stroke: Brain stimulation to enhance recovery of function of the affected hand. *Neurorehabil. Neural Repair* **2009**, *23*, 641–656. [CrossRef]
102. Chen, J.L.; Schipani, A.; Schuch, C.P.; Lam, H.; Swardfager, W.; Thiel, A.; Edwards, J.D. Does cathodal vs. sham transcranial direct current stimulation over contralesional motor cortex enhance upper limb motor recovery post-stroke? A systematic review and meta-analysis. *Front. Neurol.* **2021**, *12*, 626021. [CrossRef] [PubMed]
103. Kang, N.; Weingart, A.; Cauraugh, J.H. Transcranial direct current stimulation and suppression of contralesional primary motor cortex post-stroke: A systematic review and meta-analysis. *Brain Inj.* **2018**, *32*, 1063–1070. [CrossRef] [PubMed]
104. Lee, S.H.; Kim, W.S.; Park, J.; Kim, J.; Paik, N.J. Effects of anodal transcranial direct current stimulation over the contralesional hemisphere on motor recovery in subacute stroke patients with severe upper extremity hemiparesis: Study protocol for a randomized controlled trial. *Medicine (Baltimore)* **2020**, *99*, e19495. [CrossRef] [PubMed]
105. Chhatbar, P.Y.; Ramakrishnan, V.; Kautz, S.; George, M.S.; Adams, R.J.; Feng, W. Transcranial direct current stimulation post-stroke upper extremity motor recovery studies exhibit a dose-response relationship. *Brain Stimul.* **2016**, *9*, 16–26. [CrossRef]
106. Liao, W.W.; Chiang, W.C.; Lin, K.C.; Wu, C.Y.; Liu, C.T.; Hsieh, Y.W.; Lin, Y.C.; Chen, C.L. Timing-dependent effects of transcranial direct current stimulation with mirror therapy on daily function and motor control in chronic stroke: A randomized controlled pilot study. *J. Neuroeng. Rehabil.* **2020**, *17*, 101. [CrossRef]
107. Melendez-Calderon, A.; Rodrigues, E.; Thielbar, K.; Patton, J.L. Movement therapy without moving—First results on isometric movement training for post-stroke rehabilitation of arm function. *IEEE Int. Conf. Rehabil. Robot.* **2017**, 106–110.
108. Friedman, N.; Chan, V.; Reinkensmeyer, A.N.; Beroukhim, A.; Zambrano, G.J.; Bachman, M.; Reinkensmeyer, D.J. Retraining and assessing hand movement after stroke using the musicglove: Comparison with conventional hand therapy and isometric grip training. *J. Neuroeng. Rehabil.* **2014**, *11*, 76. [CrossRef]
109. Dragert, K.; Zehr, E.P. High-intensity unilateral dorsiflexor resistance training results in bilateral neuromuscular plasticity after stroke. *Exp. Brain Res.* **2013**, *225*, 93–104. [CrossRef]
110. Kim, H.J.; Kang, N.; Cauraugh, J.H. Transient changes in paretic and non-paretic isometric force control during bimanual submaximal and maximal contractions. *J. Neuroeng. Rehabil.* **2020**, *17*, 64. [CrossRef]
111. Kang, N.; Cauraugh, J.H. Bilateral movements increase sustained extensor force in the paretic arm. *Disabil. Rehabil.* **2018**, *40*, 912–916. [CrossRef]
112. Chollet, F.; Cramer, S.C.; Stinear, C.; Kappelle, L.J.; Baron, J.C.; Weiller, C.; Azouvi, P.; Hommel, M.; Sabatini, U.; Moulin, T.; et al. Pharmacological therapies in post stroke recovery: Recommendations for future clinical trials. *J. Neurol.* **2014**, *261*, 1461–1468. [CrossRef]
113. Liu, G.; Yang, X.; Xue, T.; Chen, S.; Wu, X.; Yan, Z.; Wang, Z.; Wu, D.; Chen, Z.; Wang, Z. Is fluoxetine good for subacute stroke? A meta-analysis evidenced from randomized controlled trials. *Front. Neurol.* **2021**, *12*, 633781. [CrossRef]
114. Siepmann, T.; Penzlin, A.I.; Kepplinger, J.; Illigens, B.M.; Weidner, K.; Reichmann, H.; Barlinn, K. Selective serotonin reuptake inhibitors to improve outcome in acute ischemic stroke: Possible mechanisms and clinical evidence. *Brain Behav.* **2015**, *5*, e00373. [CrossRef]
115. Hallett, M. Volitional control of movement: The physiology of free will. *Clin. Neurophysiol.* **2007**, *118*, 1179–1192. [CrossRef] [PubMed]

116. Georgopoulos, A.P.; Stefanis, C.N. Local shaping of function in the motor cortex: Motor contrast, directional tuning. *Brain Res. Rev.* **2007**, *55*, 383–389. [CrossRef] [PubMed]
117. Rodgers, H.; Bosomworth, H.; Krebs, H.I.; van Wijck, F.; Howel, D.; Wilson, N.; Aird, L.; Alvarado, N.; Andole, S.; Cohen, D.L.; et al. Robot assisted training for the upper limb after stroke (RATULS): A multicentre randomised controlled trial. *Lancet* **2019**, *394*, 51–62. [CrossRef]
118. Cohen, L. Interaction between limbs during bimanual voluntary activity. *Brain* **1970**, *93*, 259–272. [CrossRef] [PubMed]
119. Schaechter, J.D.; Perdue, K.L.; Wang, R. Structural damage to the corticospinal tract correlates with bilateral sensorimotor cortex reorganization in stroke patients. *Neuroimage* **2008**, *39*, 1370–1382. [CrossRef]
120. Schaffer, J.E.; Maenza, C.; Good, D.C.; Przybyla, A.; Sainburg, R.L. Left hemisphere damage produces deficits in predictive control of bilateral coordination. *Exp. Brain Res.* **2020**, *238*, 2733–2744. [CrossRef] [PubMed]
121. Marvel, C.L.; Morgan, O.P.; Kronemer, S.I. How the motor system integrates with working memory. *Neurosci. Biobehav. Rev.* **2019**, *102*, 184–194. [CrossRef]
122. Baddeley, A.D. Working memory: Looking back and looking forward. *Nat. Rev. Neurosci.* **2003**, *4*, 829–839. [CrossRef]
123. Baddeley, A.D.; Hitch, G.J. The phonological loop as a buffer store: An update. *Cortex* **2019**, *112*, 91–106. [CrossRef] [PubMed]
124. Whitall, J.; Waller, S.M.; Sorkin, J.D.; Forrester, L.W.; Macko, R.F.; Hanley, D.F.; Goldberg, A.P.; Luft, A. Bilateral and unilateral arm training improve motor function through differing neuroplastic mechanisms: A single-blinded randomized controlled trial. *Neurorehabil. Neural Repair* **2011**, *25*, 118–129. [CrossRef] [PubMed]
125. Winstein, C.; Varghese, R. Been there, done that, so what's next for arm and hand rehabilitation in stroke? *NeuroRehabilitation* **2018**, *43*, 3–18. [CrossRef] [PubMed]
126. Ward, N.S.; Brander, F.; Kelly, K. Intensive upper limb neurorehabilitation in chronic stroke: Outcomes from the queen square programme. *J. Neurol. Neurosurg. Psychiatry* **2019**, *90*, 498–506. [CrossRef]

MDPI
St. Alban-Anlage 66
4052 Basel
Switzerland
Tel. +41 61 683 77 34
Fax +41 61 302 89 18
www.mdpi.com

Applied Sciences Editorial Office
E-mail: applsci@mdpi.com
www.mdpi.com/journal/applsci

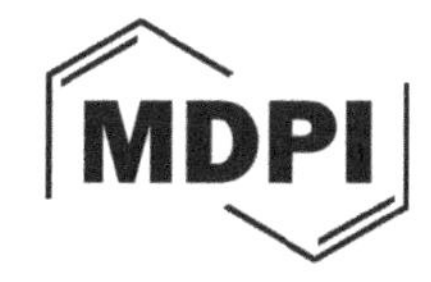

Ingram Content Group UK Ltd.
Milton Keynes UK
UKHW050246300623
424285UK00004B/64